Bedtime Stories for Adults

Over 25 Bedtime Stories to Overcome Anxiety & Insomnia, Stress Relief, and Positive Self-Healing. Help You Relaxing and Deep Sleep.

Faye Scott

© Copyright 2020 - All rights reserved.

The content contained within this book may not be reproduced, duplicated or transmitted without direct written permission from the author or the publisher.

Under no circumstances will any blame or legal responsibility be held against the publisher, or author, for any damages, reparation, or monetary loss due to the information contained within this book, either directly or indirectly.

Legal Notice:

This book is copyright protected. It is only for personal use. You cannot amend, distribute, sell, use, quote or paraphrase any part, or the content within this book, without the consent of the author or publisher.

Disclaimer Notice:

Please note the information contained within this document is for educational and entertainment purposes only. All effort has been executed to present accurate, up to date, reliable, complete information. No warranties of any kind are declared or implied. Readers acknowledge that the author is not engaged in the rendering of legal, financial, medical or professional advice. The content within this book has been derived from various sources. Please consult a licensed professional before attempting any techniques outlined in this book.

By reading this document, the reader agrees that under no circumstances is the author responsible for any losses, direct or indirect, that are incurred as a result of the use of the information contained within this document, including, but not limited to, errors, omissions, or inaccuracies.

Table of Contents

Chapter 1: To Explore the Acropolis 5

Chapter 2: The Volcano Island 11

Chapter 3: The life was so beautiful and simple 21

Chapter 4: Charli and Pam 25

Chapter 5: The Athlete 30

Chapter 6: Holiday on the Island 34

Chapter 7: The Beautiful Summer 43

Chapter 8: The Lovely Fish 50

Chapter 9: The Camping Excursion 55

Chapter 10: The Stunning World 65

Chapter 11: Alone on the Moon 70

Chapter 12: The Wisdom Search 73

Chapter 13: At the Beach 77

Chapter 14: In the Bar 81

Chapter 15: The Lemonade 87

Chapter 16: The Lunch 90

Chapter 17: The Older Adult 96

Chapter 18: The Time Travel 102

Chapter 19: A Bargain 104

Chapter 20: The Super Star 108

Chapter 21: A Hike in the Forest 114

Chapter 22: The Train Journey 118

Chapter 23: The Spirit Source 125

Chapter 24: A Mysterious Place 137

Chapter 25: Curiosity and the Cat 151

Chapter 26: A Fantasy World 154

Chapter 1: To Explore the Acropolis

Sophie and Cara have made it to Greece on their vacation, and after their resting day to catch up on all the missed sleep, they are ready to get going and finally start exploring. This day is Sophie's turn to choose what they do for the day, and she has chosen to explore the Acropolis of Athens, getting a glimpse at the past first hand.

Sophie yawned as she rolled out of bed. She was in one room of the two-room suite that Cara had insisted upon for their vacation, and so far, she loved every moment of the luxury. The flooring was a soft, plush carpet that squished so comfortably underneath her feet, almost just as invitingly as the bed had gently squished underneath her as well. The suite was overlooking the gulf to the south of Athens, and her window gave her a beautiful, breathtaking view of the bright, clear water. Across the sea, she could see land gently rolling toward the horizon as well, and there were tiny, bright sails lit up all around the water. It was a wonderful start to the morning; she told herself as she looked out at the view.

She watched for another few minutes before taking a shower in a wonderful stall, carefully tiled with beautiful marble. Getting ready in luxury was a breeze, and she was utterly relaxed as she washed the last of the soap through her hair. She was up early—her night-owl nature was really helping her out during the travels—jetlag meant that she was perfectly content being up in the daylight hours since she already normally was awake at that time, relative to her home, anyway.

Stepping out, she was greeted by a plush robe that she wrapped herself in to dry off, and she brewed a coffee using the small machine provided in her hotel room. The wondrous scent of coffee filled the air, waking her up more as it brewed. It smelled roasted and comforting—a bit of familiarity in her travels abroad, and she was thrilled to have that opportunity afforded to her in the first place. She was thrilled that her time was going to be spent enjoying the moment and actually having some peace and quiet to herself for a while. It was nice being able to take her time without waking up and immediately rushing to her computer to look over everything. It was nice being able to simply go throughout her day without being so overly concerned with everything that she was doing at any given point in time. It was enjoyable being able to go through her morning routine in leisure at her own speed.

By the time that she had finished up her coffee, she noticed that Cara had finished getting herself ready as well. She stepped out of her own room in a nice, airy blue dress that gently clung to her waist, and half of her hair tied up and back, out of her face. She wore tan strapped sandals that somehow managed to be the perfect blend of functional and attractive at the same time, and her black sunglasses were carefully perched atop her head. Her makeup was impeccably done, perfectly put on while still somehow managing to capture that natural look to it as well. She looked great. Even on vacation and even when their itinerary for the day involved walking, she still managed to look wonderful. It was a wonder she was still single, Sophie marveled as she looked on toward her friend. "You're not ready yet?" Cara asked, raising a perfectly sculpted eyebrow up in surprise.

Sophie grinned back. "I'm enjoying taking my time for a change! I'll be ready to go in a few minutes." All she really had left to do was get dressed, and she'd be good to go, too. She wasn't nearly as particular about her looks as Cara tended to be. So, while Cara sipped at her own coffee on the balcony overlooking the gulf, Sophie got ready to go. She tossed on some khaki high-waisted shorts that came just above her knees and a white chiffon top, tucked into the waistband. She was comfortable, yet functional as she also tied on her walking shoes and picked up the wide-brimmed hat that she placed atop her head. She walked out to meet Cara, waving for her to follow.

Cara stood up and put away her cup. "That looks quaint," she acknowledged with a smile.

"Thanks," Sophie said, choosing to take the comment as a compliment rather than bothering to say a word about it. She grinned and bounced as they walked down the hall together. She was brimming with excitement—heading to visit Acropolis had been one of her lifelong dreams that she had for herself, and she was finally living it! She was so happy to do so, and even though she knew that it would be crowded and nothing like it once was, there was something thrilling about going somewhere that was built nearly 2500 years ago. Though it was beginning to crumble, it was a real testament to the power of humanity, even that long ago.

Sophie was incredibly impressed with what she had seen in the books—every time she ever looked at the pictures of the ruins, it was gorgeous—tall, crumbling, and flawed, but that made it so much more awe-inspiring to view. It was made before humanity had levels and laser pointers to help them measure our angles just right. They built them before people had machines to help lift these massive behemoths of stone and marble. They were so immaculately and impeccably carved for people that only had their hands and small hand tools to work with, and she couldn't help but be fascinated with them. She loved being able to explore them, to learn about the world around her, and to learn how to better begin to relate to how people used to live.

Cara might not enjoy exploring around as much as the shopping and the sightseeing, but for Sophie, being able to see just how humanity used to live was so worth every moment of travel that came with it. She didn't particularly enjoy flying, but getting to go around all of the different historical sites gave her a great perspective over everything and everyone involved.

Stepping outside of the hotel had them immediately hit with warm, humid air that smelled of the beach and of promise for a day of fantastic exploration and sightseeing. It smelled of excitement and of being able to meet those lifelong goals once and for all, and Sophie was entirely ready to throw herself into it all. Even Cara, who was typically uninterested in such events and fun, had a smile on her face as they walked out. Even though Cara had a tendency to be very set in her ways, she had a huge soft spot for making sure that her dear friend was happy, and this day was no exception to that matter. She was willing to put on a happy face to go through everything with her friend if it meant seeing Sophie's dream come true.

"Did you know that Acropolis is referred to as the crowning jewel of Greece, and it is the birthplace of democracy?" Sophie practically squealed as she walked through the path. "It's such an important site! AND, even though it was damaged, it is still there for us to see now."

"Really?" Cara asked in return. It was hard not to feel excited when she watched Sophie bubbling over the words that were being said. She grinned back at her friend. It was always pleasant to see just how worked up Sophie would get when she was talking about something she loved. "What happened to it anyway?"

"What, with the damage?"

"Yeah. It's pretty broken down now, isn't it?" Cara replied as they made their way to the site.

"It is! So back during the Morean War, the war between the Turkish and Venice, Acropolis held the gunpowder that they would use. But, during a battle in 1687, the Parthenon, the main building that everyone thinks about when they're thinking of the Acropolis, was hit with a cannonball. When that happened, it kind of all blew up! And now, it has that broken down look that it had. But, there's more to Acropolis than just the Parthenon, too. It was a great big citadel built atop a big hill. It was called acropolis because it is so high—did you know that acro means extreme or high, while polis means city? It's high up in the city, and the one in Athens is the most popular." Sophie was bouncing along with every step as she talked away. She knew her Greek history and mythology and was not afraid to show it off.

"Wow, that's... A lot of a lot!" Cara said, patting Sophie on the shoulder. "But I'm really excited to go see everything. It should look great."

"Me too!" Sophie squealed.

It didn't take them long to arrive at the location where their tour bus would pick them up, and they waited among the small crowd of people, happily chatting. The Acropolis was in the center of the city, overlooking everything around it. It had once been the home of some of the most important parts of the city, dedicated to Athena, the patron of the city, and it was an incredibly popular tourist site year-round. This meant two things: One, that they would have to be around lots of people, but two, that they would be able to get to the site without having to walk all across Athens.

The bus was filled up, and before they knew it, they were being addressed by the tour guide. He was a tall, thin young man with beautiful olive skin. His hair was trimmed at the sides and slicked back, and his face was impeccably sculpted. His eyes were kind as he talked to them, and he appeared to be genuinely passionate about his heritage as he spoke to them.

"Ooh, look at the eye candy," Cara said, nudging Sophie on the bus with a sly smile on her face and giggling.

Sophie looked at her with a scandalized expression. "Shh!!" she shushed her friend, giggling quietly as well. Cara was not wrong—he was a very handsome man, and even better, he was telling them all about everything that they would be learning about on the tour. But, what he had to say was mostly just the same details that Sophie had parroted about the entire walk to the stop. He mentioned the history and what they could expect, as well as some rules that they would all have to follow to ensure that everything went smoothly.

"The hill was picked out," he said through his Greek accent, "Primarily because of the fact that it sat so high up. It was the area where the locals settled down to live, and the rock at the top was deemed where the ruler would live. It was not until later that it gained recognition as being associated with the goddess Athena, and it was not until the 8th century. Athena gained her own temple on the northeastern side of the hill." He looked around the tour bus, seeing that most of the people were only mildly interested at best. "But, the Parthenon is the most popular of all. It has withstood over the centuries, surviving fire, earthquakes, wars, and even explosions while still standing. It was once a powerful symbol of religion and culture of Athens, and today, it still endures, showing the true perseverance of the Greek people and of the Athenians themselves."

Sophie grinned at the man, glad to hear someone else sharing her passion for the history of such a magnificent building, but she was not interested in approaching him, even with Cara's incessant nudging. Yes, he was good looking, but she didn't really want to go through the hassle of an international fling, even if it were just a temporary ordeal. That didn't sound particularly appealing to her, even if they both shared a certain appreciation for the Greek culture.

Before long, they had arrived. The bus slowly squealed to a stop, and they all unloaded, one by one, to get off the bus. Then, Sophie got her first glance of it all. They were down toward the bottom of the rocky wall that built up the city. They were in for plenty of walking, but still, the sight was breathtaking. Against the blue sky, she could see the buildings, all aligned. The Parthenon's stark white walls and pillars clashed against the sky, and she could see that the line was already building up.

"This," the tour guide called out, pointing to the entrance to the area, "is the path to the center of it all. It is here that you will be able to follow the path that thousands of years ago, the ancient people of Athens walked when they entered this sacred area. This is the road to the Parthenon, to the altar of Athena, and more. As you enter, remember to remain respectful. This area is ancient—it deserves the respect that you would have in any ancient relic. It is a part of my people's history, and if you cannot honor the rules. Where you are standing right now is the gate to the Acropolis, the Propylaia. It was here that people were able to enter, and in order to pass through, in the time when this sanctuary was dedicated to the great Athena, only certain people were allowed to enter. You must take nothing, and you must leave nothing but your footsteps behind in this great, sacred place. Now, are you ready?"

The group of people in the tour all gave a weak cheer and chuckle, and off they went into the site. It was beautiful, Sophie marveled as they finally took their first steps in. The stones were surprisingly lightly colored underneath her feet, and she looked up at the eight massive pillars supporting the beam that undoubtedly once made up the building's roof in front of her. Sophie was practically bouncing in excitement as they stood outside under the sun—she was thrilled to see everything in front of her, and she was ready to dive in. Of course, the tour had different plans.

As they toured the structures, they slowly traveled from ruin to ruin. Their tour guide was happy to explain to them everything that they would be doing and why he loved each and every building. He was quick to provide information about every single building.

The first stop was the Erechtheion, a temple located in the northern part of the Acropolis. As Sophie gazed upon the building's crumbling walls and the strange sculptures of women on one end, she listened closely. "The Porch of the Maidens," her tour guide begun, "Was added there to hide the beam that supports the southwest corner of the building. Due to budgeting constraints after the beginning of the Peloponnesian War, the building's size was cut, and as such, they had to find a way to disguise the pillar. Thus, the caryatids were built to create something beautiful to view and look at them!" All six women stood there, balancing the roof of the building on their heads, and yet, each and every single one looked graceful.

Before long, they had moved on to the Temple of Athena Nike. The massive temple stood tall on the stretch of land. It was built to provide a place to honor Athena Nike, the goddess of victory. It was a beautiful temple, complete with a beautiful carving of Athena herself trying to adjust the strap of a sandal.

They made it through several of the buildings, but the last one that they approached was the one that Sophie had been looking forward to the most: The Parthenon. "The Parthenon was created," the tour guide begun, "Primarily to provide people with a place to gather. It was the hubbub for all religious life in Athens, and the temple itself, built by Pericles, was believed to represent the power, lavish culture, and wealth that Athens enjoyed during the time. Today, it has remained one of the largest and most recognizable buildings that exist. It was eventually overtaken by the Byzantines after their conquering of Greece and was turned into a church. Then, again, it was converted when another empire, the Ottomans, took over Athens. It was converted then into a mosque. However, upon the war in 1687, the building was detonated when a cannonball from the Christian Holy League, attempting to reclaim their land, hit the ammunition depot and caused a detonation."

"Oh, so you were right!" Cara said with a grin.

"Shh!" Sophie hushed her as she marveled at the building. Though in ruins now, it was still magnificent to look on to. It was huge—a massive testament to human ability and skill, and something about it was absolutely amazing to behold. Her heart was happy—she had finally managed to check another item off her bucket list.

Chapter 2: The Volcano Island

You can have a sense of finding yourself walking through a museum as you walk through that Museum so you can hear the way that your footsteps echo off. The walls you can listen to doors being opened and closing. The way the sounds of the doors echo through the corridor and down into each room and Museum. While you walk around the museum, so you notice that everyone is beginning to leave. But the museum is starting to close for the night. You're here to keep an eye on the paintings the statues when everyone's gone home. So you walk around checking that everyone's leaving the museum. While you walk around, you notice different sculptures, different paintings, large paintings, smaller paintings. You hear the different doors being closed as different rooms are empty of people until eventually, all the customers have left. Then the other staff leave and leave you to keep an eye on the museum yourself. After the last person has left and the front door has been closed, so you go and sit down. Somewhere in one of the rooms and the idea is that you'll sit down in a room. Then every 15 20 minutes, you'll stand up and walk to another room and sit down there for a while.

Just doing the rounds so that you're in each room as the night goes on being still being able to listen in case there are any sounds in the museum. As you sit in one of the rooms, so you hear some sounds. You decide to go and investigate, and what you find in one of the rooms is the sound of tribal drums. Then you can't figure out where that sound is coming from, and then you notice that some of the statues start to come alive. Then one of the icons comes over to you, and you're a little surprised by this. The figure comes over to you and says that your help is needed that you need to find a lost gem, a gem that belongs to one of the figures in the museum. Until that gem is placed back in the figure, things can't settle, and you don't understand exactly why or what they mean, but the way that they describe this makes you think you've got to go and help in some way. You think it's got to be more exciting than just sitting in one room or another in silence.

So, you ask what it is you need to do, and the statue looks over at a painting. You walk over to that painting, and as you get to that painting, you gaze into it. You notice how large that art is that the picture is taller than you are and at least twice as wide. You look into that painting, and you can see it's a painting of a volcanic island. A volcanic island containing a forest as you don't know what you're supposed to do, then notice there seems to be something unusual about this painting. There appears to be a slight shimmer to the art, so you reach out with your hand and gently put your fingertips onto the artwork. As you place your fingers onto the painting, your hand starts to go through the canvas, and it feels like your hand is gently lowered into some freshwater. You can contact the surface tension around your fingers. You can think that moving up your fingers to your palm of your hand and then keeping it in your hand.

You can feel it moving to your wrist and then slowly tickling and tingling as it moves up your arm as you push your hair and into the painting. After your arm is in the picture, so you step in and follow it. She finds yourself in that painting on the volcanic island, and you can hear a thunderstorm start to rage here lashes of rain. You begin to get soaking wet see run into the forest and as you run into the woods. You notice how the rain changes you can now hear that rain falling on the leaves above you listen to it bouncing on those leaves here the thwap sound as each large raindrop hits the large leaves. You're relatively dry inside this forest with such dense forest around you, and you can hear the rumble of thunder. Notice shards of light appear from above as the thunder rolls and lightning flashes. You walk through this forest and feel lucky that it's quite warm here as you walk further into the woods.

You start to dry off while being protected from that rain protected from the raging storm. You continue walking further through the forest you don't yet know what you're looking for how you're going to find this gem. Where this gem is and as you continue walking through the forest, so from time to time, you reach out and touch the bark of trees fill that at your fingertips. You can feel the third of each footstep on the ground, the dull thud as the sound gets absorbed by all the woodland you can hear that storm above hear that heavy rain on the leaves. You continue walking more profoundly and more in-depth, and as you keep walking, you don't know where you're going. And there just seems to be a bit more of a path on the route that you're taking. You recall what this picture looked like before you stepped into it. So you try to remember that in your mind, almost like a map trying to work out where you must have appeared. Where you must be now, you know that you're on a volcanic island. You're currently not walking uphill or downhill. You know you're not stepping up towards the center of the island or down directly towards the coast. You must be walking across the island, which means at some point you'll start walking down.

But for now, you're just walking through the forest and after some time of walking through the woods. You start here a bit more wind coming from in front of you, and you realize you must be approaching the edge of the woods. Although most of the rain isn't making its way to you and isn't falling on you, he's being blocked by the canopy above. You're aware that you're going to need to keep dry when you get out the other side. So what you start doing is collecting some of the big leaves around you. You begin collecting some more significant bits of wood, and on some trees, they have bark, which you can cut at the top. Then you can peel it off in strips, almost like a rope. So you do that and get yourself a load of pieces of bark then as you approach the far side of the forest. You start to see some light again, and you know that warm, and yet there's some light because above the storm. The Sun hasn't set yet, and so you clear the forest walking back out into the rain, you see that you're near the edge of a cliff. So you decide to set up a camp here.

You need to set something up that can just keep you dry and protected. You decide you'll continue your search when the storm has passed see make a pyramid with the more significant bits of wood you tie it all into place with bark bits. You weave in the leaves tie some of them into place, creating a watertight shelter. You place some of the other leaves inside, and then you cruel inside your tent and relax down. While you relax down, so the storm rages on, let's light up with lightning, you can hear the rumble of thunder and understand the large raindrops hitting the ground around you hitting your makeshift tent. Now you're in the dry and sitting down; you feel so relaxed. You find the sounds calming relaxing you find their peaceful they make your mind just want to drift and wander, and from where you are, you're looking out off a cliff over the sea. You can see that seas are quite rough at the moment much of its clouded by the falling rain. So while you sit in your makeshift tent, your eyes begin to close. As your eyes start to close, so your mind starts to drift and dream, and you drift and dream and float back through time in your account. You begin to have this sense have almost been like a bad of just flying over the ocean seeing this clear blue sea seeing comfortable rolling waves.

You drift back through time, and you have a sense of wonder about this island. You're on what the island was like before it was an island how did it become this volcanic island, drifting and floating through the time you have this sense of underwater deep down. A volcano is gently erupting lava is spewing out crackling and popping as it reacts with the water glowing red in the deep blue sea as it gradually builds up. This island from deep under the ocean building. This island up higher and higher towards the surface, and you watch in your mind's eye. As that continues at a steady pace and then occasionally, a more massive eruption happens. Under the sea and the island gets a growth spurt, and then after thousands of years, Ireland begins to get nearer to the surface. Then gradually, the whole time, the land over the magma is shifting slightly. The island is gently elongating until, eventually, one day, the tiniest island appeared above the waves. Initially, just creating some ripples on the surface where it was just below the surface most of the time and only at low tide would it be just above the surface.

Until one day, there was this tiny island. Then the volcano continued erupting and grooved 1-meter square island to meet a square island 4-meter square Island 8-meter square Island 16-meter square Island. It started growing exponentially while the whole time, the island was moving. While the magma was remaining in the same place. After a while, there was this vast black island above the surface of the water with nothing. But black rock and then as time continued, so the Earth's plates continued to move. Thus the magma was creating other islands elsewhere and no longer producing this island. Then as thousands of years continue to pass, random seeds are blown. In the breeze around the earth would find themselves caught on the island and then one-day thousands and thousands of years ago the tiniest little sprout of green started growing on the island followed by another and another. Until the island started turning from black to green and then as even more time passed little sprouts of trees began springing up. Suddenly these trees started growing taller and taller and over hundreds of years. They expanded into tall forests encircling the volcanic island.

The water crashed against the island, creating areas of beaches and the other regions of cliffs. Then as thousands of years continued, some life would find its way to the island floating on branches and leaves from other places. The occasionally lost bird landing and making the island their home, and some would survive and find others. Then create more, and others would be the only one of their kind would make the island their home for their life. As thousands and thousands of years passed trees and plants, multiple generations of experience exist on the island. They have lived on the island, then you float around and drift around like a bird. In the sky, they are finding it fascinating looking down on this island, watching the evolution of this island from when it was just forming on the ocean surf on the bottom of the ocean watching. As it grew up to lore until I broke the surface of the ocean became an island that you see now that you recognize as being like the island. You're currently camping on, and your mind drift wanders seas the island.

The most beautiful calm sea with the most beautiful sky as your attention then draws back to the fact you're in a tent. You're in a makeshift shelter on the edge of a cliff gazing out over the ocean with the storm raging around you. And you look out of the tent you see the heavy rain falling in front of you. You hear the sound of the rain on your makeshift shelter. You can see the rough sea and the lighting and darkening of the clouds as lightning rumbles through the sky and as you continue to watch. So you notice how that rumbling thunder how that storm seems to be weakening. You can then see how rain is falling over the ocean and no longer falling over you as you continue watching so as that storm moves further out to sea as that storm passes by towards. The horizon and you watch the way the Lightning dances in the clouds make the tops of the clouds glow and flash and flicker before a low rumbling of thunder reaches your ears. You notice how the sea below you appears to be calming as that storm moves. Further away and after some time you notice the storm has moved far enough away that you can see some glass sky you can see some cloudless sky.

You can notice the red hue to the sky, and you know that somewhere behind that storm, a Sun is setting as you watch that red hue dimming down. You sit there gazing out to sea, watching that storm at night until eventually, the rumbles get so quiet. You can barely make them out, and yet you can still see on her eyes. The way that storms in those clouds high up into the air as lightning dancing flashing and flickering making those clouds glow with white light, almost like a light machine in a party flickering that white light through those clouds. As hours continue to pass, that storm gets more distant until you see that it's almost entirely over the horizon. You can see at the same time the Sun is practically wholly set. There's just the faintest orange glow on the horizon. As the Sunsets over the background and the storm pass by, the sky ends up a cloudless sky, the air smells. So fresh and clean and bright, you can start to hear sounds around you of wildlife. In the forest, so relaxing, then you start gazing up at the sky, gazing up at all the stars seeing more appearing as the light disappears.

And as your eyes begin to get used to the dark and you just gaze up comfortably in awe at the sky feeling—a sense of how small you are when looking at such a blanket of beauty. As you gaze up at that sky, you notice a meteor shower happening. You start to see streaks of light flashing across the sky, in all directions looking like they're coming from a constellation of Leo and you watch as that happens from that constellation. As you watch those meteors flashing across the sky, you feel like you can hear the fizzing and popping. And you know it must be in your mind because you know there's no time for the sound to have reached your ears. Yet because they'd be burning up high in the atmosphere and again, you feel like you can hear the fizzing and popping. You notice some of them are slightly different colors to white; you even have this sense like you can smell the meteorites. As if they're landing near you almost like the smell of a sparkler. But again, you know that just must be in your mind. Because of how intensely focused you are on the beauty of this, how dark it is be getting here.

While it's getting darker and darker here so you realize you can see the Stars meet yours brighter than you ever could before in your life. You get so drawn into the experience you almost forget that you stepped into a painting. This is all taking place inside an art because you should be in the museum. Yet this all feels so real to you, almost like this is real, it all feels. So real to you, it doesn't feel like you're in a painting, not that you'd know what being in a picture would feel like. So as you continue to gaze up at the sky gaze over the sea, which now looks jet-black, you decide it's time to close your eyes. Rest for the night you'll try and find the gym in the morning so you take a moment to settle down and your makeshift you close your eyes. You fool asleep, and while you sleep, you start to hear the sound of water being pushed aside like always driving through the water. You feel so comfortable that you feel like you're resting and sleeping in that early, dozy state where you can feel asleep.

Yet feel awake at the same time, and you feel so relaxed, and then you start to feel the warmth of the Sun on your face. So you listen to that water around you just the subtle slightest lapping of the water around you the feeling of the warmth of the Sun on you the pushing sound of the water almost like was gently pushing through the water. Then after a few moments, you start to come around, and you begin to open your eyes. You realize you've been sleeping on the back of a giant turtle, and you feel perfectly fine and calm and curious. You start looking around you, and in every direction, all you see is the smoothest most beautiful turquoise e blue water that leads to a turquoise e blue sky. The color of the water and the sky's color are so similar you can't tell the difference between the rain. The air you can't see where the horizon is, you can't know where the sea ends and where the sky begins. You look in front of you, and you look all around you. You look behind you and feel that turtle beneath you the smoothness of its shell as it continues to swim through the ocean.

As it swims so, it could almost be staying stationary because nothing around you changes. You can't see anything you're heading toward or anything you're heading away from you can't see anything to the left or the right of you or anywhere else around you. The perfect blue just surrounds you. After a while, the turtle lowers its head and starts to dive beneath the water's surface. As you dive beneath the water's surface on the turtle's back, you hold on as it falls. You notice straight away that you can breathe underwater just as quickly as you can on the surface. That the turtle is breathing just as soon as it does on the surface. You can hear bubbles of air with each out-breath coming from you coming from the turtle. You can feel the water on you as you push through that water diving deeper and deeper. As you dive deeper, the bottom of the ocean begins to come into view. You can see fish just going about their everyday lives; you can see how seaweed is swaying and moving under the surface of the water. You don't know where you're diving too, or you know as you seem to be diving deeper.

After some time you are diving deeper and deeper, the turtle levels off. It starts to follow what looks almost like a path of pure white sand between two cliffs. It's an extensive path, and after a while, two mermaids appear either side. As if to escort you somewhere and they're swimming along silently either side of the turtle. As you swim on that turtle's back following this path, unsure exactly where you're going, just feeling curious about the experience. Then after you turn a couple of corners so the sides give way to an open plane of whites and whites and that appears to have waves built into it that has rippled across that sand and off. In the distance, you see what looks like a Crystal Palace. You notice that the turtle is swimming towards that palace and that these mermaids are escorting you towards. This palace and all the fish go about their lives but move out your way as you're heading towards that Palace. Then after a while, you find yourself entering into the palace entrance when you follow along corridor being escorted by these mermaids. At the end of a long corridor is a massive door, and Toomer people open the door stand aside. As the mermaids and the turtle in yourself' pass through into a vast chamber.

The high ceiling chandeliers light glistening and reflecting everywhere merpeople are standing down both sides what looks like a king and queen on Thrones. The turtle lands on the ground, allowing it's headed the mermaids to swim off and join the other people you climb off the turtle's back. You walk your way through the water, finding it easy and effortless to walk through the water, finding it more comfortable than you expected. You walk through the water and stand in front of the king and queen. They tell you that what you seek is rooted in the valley at the end of a cave, and only two legs can find it. You don't know what this means, but you sure this must be something to do with what you're searching for they say to return. After you've got what you seek, so you go back to the turtle climb back onto the turtle shell, the turtle raises its head moves its fins pushing off. The ground is turning around swimming back out of the chamber down the corridor and out of the palace. The turtle swims around the outside of the palace and starts swimming along behind the palace away from the castle.

Further and further until eventually, there appears to be a cliff, and the turtle dive straight down into that cliff going deeper and deeper, under the surface of the ocean, swimming down deeper and further and further and more profound. As the water gets darker and darker, then you notice as you're swimming down deeper. Further, how everything seems to get quieter how it's interesting that time seems to almost standing still underwater, everything seems to be in slow motion. You swim down deeper and deeper, and after some time, you find you can barely see in front. Then you notice that there's some ground approaching, then the turtle follows that ground and swims along and finds the entrance to a cave. You realize you can barely see now there's no way you're going to be able to see in the cave. You start to focus on the solution that you want some light you want to be able to see inside the cave. You start focusing on that solution. You focus on what it is you want as you're focusing on what it is you want. So you find that you can see little green lights starting to flicker all around you, getting closer and brighter and brighter and closer.

You notice a shoal of fish starts to form around you, and the turtle below you above you to leave to the right behind you of bioluminescent fish. They're swimming on the spot or all around you lighting up where you are almost turning the whole of you into a giant torch. Then you think about going into the cave, and the turtle starts into the cave. As the turtle does so, the fish keep pace with you and swims in with you. You notice the green glow of the fish on the walls—the cave on the floor of the cave, the roof of the cave swimming into that cave. You swim more profound and deeper into that cave. I'm sure what you're going to discover is swimming more intelligent and more in-depth.

Further and further, and then you start to notice something in front of you, it looks like off in the distance is a wooden door. You arrive at that wooden door you get off of the turtle you knock on the door and hear the underwater knock you then knock in another location. You try and find a way through the door. You can't find any easy, obvious way, and then you see on the ground two marks that almost looked like footprints.

So, you put one foot on one mark one foot on another score, and nothing happens. You bounce around a bit, and still, nothing happens, then you see a mark on the wall on one side and the other side. You reach out, and you put your hands on those marks, and you push in all four directions. At the same time, pushing down with both legs and pushing on the wall with both hands. Then you hear a clunk and notice how that wooden door slides aside. You enter through the wooden door and find yourself inside a large chamber. In the center of that chamber and you notice the way that light seems to be coming from somewhere almost like light is perhaps channeled from the surface. Um, how through the cave-in two beams straight onto that gem, and you see the way that gem is lit up by those beams of light. You pick the gem up off the pedestal notice. It's the most beautiful gem you've ever seen, and you feel that in your fingers. In the palm of your hand, you feel the weight of that you roll it around. Your fingers gently and slowly, and as you do so down into the ground, you can hear the rumble of rock.

As the pedestal lowers and as you notice a little chamber at the back, opening up as a rock door slides aside. She walked the end of the house when he finds a scroll, and you pick up that scroll. Decide to take the scroll and the gem back with you, and you head back you get back on the turtle. You start to swim out of the cave with all those fish surrounding you swim out of the cave. When you get outside the cave, the fish start following you up through the darkness than when you reach a point where the light allows the fish to disperse and swim away. The turtle continues swimming up and then around and heads round to the entrance to the palace. It floats its way into the castle, swims back to the central room lands on the ground. You walk to the king and queen, and you say you found the gem, and they say you can keep the gem. You say you also found the scroll, and they tell you it's a scroll that they've known the existence of but have never been able to get. Yet it's a scroll that can maintain peace across the land, and you hand over the parchment. They thank you for that, and they know that the knowledge the wisdom can be taught to the people of the land taught far and wide to bring peace and comfort.

You walk back to the turtle climb back on the turtle and swim out of the palace swim back out across vast open white flats of sand finding your way. And back to the surface and then when you reach the surface, you notice that nothing has changed. You still can't see anything in any direction. There's still just this beautiful blue, the slightest movement of the water. The sound almost like oars of the turtle swimming through that water. You rest on the back of that turtle as it swims through the water. While it swims through the water, so you rest your cheek on the end of the turtle, you can feel the back of that turtle against your cheek. You can feel the warmth of the Sun. You feel comfort relaxation, and you feel yourself beginning to drift comfortably asleep as you drift comfortably asleep so you can hear in the background the slight sound of the water. The sound of the turtle swimming feels the warmth of the Sun feels your gentle breathing. Gradually the sour begin to fade away; slowly, it all starts to fade away.

You find yourself beginning to hear Siebert beginning to listen to a louder see against the shore in the cliff starting to look. But other sounds in the forest feeling a breeze on your skin. You find yourself back in that tent again in that makeshift tent gazing out off that cliff over the ocean seeing the blue sky, seeing the Sun rising aware that storm has long passed feeling the breeze on your face. You surprised yourself by finding that the gem is in your hand and that somehow that experience on the turtle even though you feel like you fell asleep. It was a dream that was somehow real, but then you're unsure about how real because you're already inside a painting, you fell asleep in art and ends up in the sea on a turtle. You don't question it something feels comfortable about it. So you take that gem you leave your camp, and you head off into the forest, starting to make your way back to where you came from. You walk through the woods, unsure exactly where you're going to go or how you're supposed to get back out of the painting.

You walk through the forest, just trusting yourself walking through our woods, hearing the sounds in the woods the relaxing sounds in the woods the sounds of each footstep. The feeling of breeze the sounds of rustling leaves as the wind blows in the trees finding your way through the woods. Then after a while, you find your way out the other side of the forest, and you see a tree that seems fuzzy. You walk over to that old fuzzy tree you go to touch the bark of that fuzzy tree and find your hand starts going into the tree. So, you put your hand in your arm in, and eventually, you take a step through that tree. You find yourself back in the museum, and you show the living statue of the gem. The statue says that's the gem that was needed the treasure that will help them all to finally sleep and rest that will help everything go back to the way. It should be, and the statue explains why that gem so important and walks you round to a specific statue. In the head of that statue is a gap where this gem should be, then you place that gem in the difference in that statue.

As you do so, the other statue starts walking away back to where it's supposed to be stood. Before it's reached where it's supposed to be held, it grinds to a halt and stops in a standing position, and everything goes silent. You walk back to that painting, and you touch the art, and it's just a typical painting of a volcanic island. You're unsure what to make of your experience as your shift comes to an end. You go home in the morning and pondering. Your knowledge and the meaning of your experience, you go to bed and as you go to bed. So, you fall asleep, and as you fall asleep, so you drift and dream you hear tribal drums. You find yourself on that volcanic island sitting in your makeshift tent, gazing out over the ocean aware that when you fall asleep here in this tent. You'll find yourself awakening on the back of that turtle, awaiting whatever adventures happen next.

Chapter 3: The life was so beautiful and simple

There was a seahorse named Mike, who lived at the bottom of the sea with his pals. The life there was so beautiful and simple. They could start their day by eating breakfast, going to school, doing schoolwork, having some time to play, doing house chores, grabbing dinner, and getting ready for bed. That

was the typical routine, day in and day out. Life there was excellent, but the fish still thought something was missing. The fish could go out playing, and Mike would join the games, as well. After some time, the fish realized that their time playing was limited. The fish could give Mike homework to do for him as he played. Mike was always encouraged to do his homework and not play with the fish who liked playing more than doing the assignments. After some time, the seahorse started being reluctant to help the fish on his homework, but the fish wanted to be assisted, whatever it took.

Mike felt lonely because he influenced his other friends not to play with him. He was always alone because the fish and his friends considered him a bookworm and did not want to associate with him. He started coming closer to them, but nothing changed about that. He was doing this just to have his friends back again, but they still mistreated him and made him feel worthless.

"Go and study; don't play with us. You are not our type," said the fish to Mike, who left them with sadness.

Mike felt like he had lost all his friends and was going to be just alone with his books. This action from the fish and his friends affected him, but he had no option but to accept what had happened. In school, the fish told everyone how the seahorse was mean at home, and he doesn't deserve any friends. Mike kept calm and could do his stuff all alone now that he realized no one was on his side. They had a contest in their school, and Mike was one of the participants.

All the other competitors had support from their classmates and friends, but for the seahorse, no one was on his side. He trained alone after everyone else

had finished training. He used to train alone while his sister watched him and corrected him.

"You can do it, brother; you are the best," her sister told him.

Her sister was his number one fan and could always cheer for him when they are training in the house. On the other hand, the fish had support from his friends, and he was the main competitor against Mike. They used to frustrate Mike on where to train until he decided to prepare at home, and they had nothing to put against him. Everyone in school knew there was a competition between Mike and the fish. Time was moving, and the contest was after the students were done with their exams.

When the exams were finished, the results came out, and the seahorse was the first in their class, and as always, the fish and the other friends felt jealous about his position. He could say nothing but just kept silent on what they said about him.

"You can beat us when it comes to education, but not when it comes to the contest," said the fish.

Days passed, and the competition day was coming to a close, and everyone was full of joy waiting for that day. The crew of the fish had a lot of confidence that they knew winning would be on their side. Preparations were getting more stringent, and the seahorse felt terrified due to lack of friends and feared how he would be frustrated during the competitions. As always, his small sister would encourage him to put more effort and not be scared of his opponents. He designed his costumes and was ready for the contest; he

was so much into singing that he felt he could win it when the day came.

Mike could sing for his family and entertain them during dinner. He had such a beautiful tonal variation that all his family members rallied behind him and encouraged him. He could always sing everywhere he was while walking, taking a shower, or eating. So many people in his neighborhood envied his voice. The fish could hear him sing and felt so bad and wanted to do anything possible to prevent Mike from performing.

They had a few days for them to present their talents. Everyone was eagerly waiting, including the parents and the teachers who knew how stiff the competition was going to be.

"The winner will get a scholarship and free education," said the headteacher.

Everyone cheered as this was an exciting offer and the winner was going to study for free. So many people rallied behind the fish as they had seen him training, but no one had seen the seahorse do his training. The stage was decorated, and everything was put in place on that eve of the competition day. Mike left school for home, and on his way, he met the bully fish with his friends.

"I will defeat you, and I will be the one to take the awards," said the fish.

Upon reaching home, Mike rehearsed as always and sang a very emotional song to his family, and everybody cheered him in the house. He told his mother how he was facing frustrations at school, and he wasn't even sure about the competition.

"You can do it, son. We are all your biggest fans, and tomorrow, we shall come and cheer you," his mother said.

He prepared his costumes, and to his surprise, his dad bought him new shoes, and this boosted his morale for the competition. He was so happy, and before he slept, his sister held his hand and prayed for him. This was so beautiful that he slept feeling so loved, having a lot of support from his family.

"Wake up! It's your day today, big brother," said his sister.

Her mum had already prepared everything for him, and he woke up and prepared himself for the challenge ahead. After eating breakfast and putting on his costume, he left for school together with his family. He felt so happy, and they had prayed together as a family, and this gave him some extra confidence in the competition.

"Son, this is the best occasion to show everyone how special you are," said his dad.

Mike smiled and felt he could not let down his family members. Everyone was already coming to the hall, and the participants were going backstage to wait for their time. A lot of guests were there, and the room was full of many people.

"This is my day, and I have to do my best," said Mike to himself.

The competition started, and a lot of people were waiting for the fish and the

seahorse on stage, as they were the most significant opponents for the show that day.

"On stage, we have Mike," said the emcee.

The whole crowd jumped in cheers as others just heckled him. Then when he came on stage, everyone else went silent just waiting to hear him perform. There was so much silence in the hall that a pin drop could be heard. As he started singing, his mum stood and shouted, "that's my boy! Go, son, you can make it."

It was so inspiring that everyone else clapped at Mike, who was now winning people's hearts with his beautiful voice. He sang well that by the time he left the stage, everyone was chanting his name, suggesting he did a great job. His whole family went and congratulated him for the high performance; he was so happy and went to watch his friend perform. The fish came on stage, and his performance, too, was so outstanding that people thought he outshined Mike only for him to mess while playing.

He felt so bad that he left the stage crying and bitter about himself. Just as he went to change his costumes, the first person to embrace him was Mike, who encouraged him and told him he did well. He felt like he was playing games with him and pushed him away.

"Leave me alone; you are just making fun of me," said the fish to Mike.

All the other performances were done, and it was now time for the results, and everyone felt so tensed about the outcome. The results were read up to

position three, and it was time to announce the second and first positions. The room was so silent, and then the second place was given to Mike. The whole place was full of screams as they knew that the fish was the winner.

"Sorry, everyone. There is a mistake," said the emcee.

In first place was Mike, whose family jumped up in joy and told him he was great as they had told him. The whole place heckled him, but some people cheered his victory, which was very honest. Mike came on stage and gave out his speech, which was very inspiring. He talked about his frustrations from his friends, but he still pushed on not to be held back by anything. Mike said he had forgiven the fish for everything that he did against him. He went ahead to tell them that he would share his awards with the fish, which was in tears after everything he said. The whole crowd felt moved by what Mike said, and they started cheering at him once again. The competition was successful, and the two friends were brought back together again. They hugged each other tightly. The story tells us to always be there for our friends, whatever the situation was. What goes around will always come back around.

Chapter 4: Charli and Pam

Charli and Pam were happily married and were going out tonight. It was their anniversary, and they were still just as much in love and infatuated with each other as the day that they met. They were two very lucky people, as they had learned over the years that many of the people they knew from their college days had also married but were now divorced. This, they attributed to the fact that they had always meditated together since the beginning, and that meant that they were two very relaxed people. They were, however, looking for something new to do and decided to take a trip to Hawaii.

They flew over to Oahu and stayed in a rental overlooking the Ala Wai. One night, they went out to a Luau. Neither of them had ever been to one before, and they had a blast together. They stayed all the way until the end and then decided to take a walk. They went back to their rental car and got a pair of flashlights they had seen in the trunk. The party was on the beach but far down the coast and away from the main part of town. The beach was bordered by a deep and lush forest of Hawaiian foliage.

They looked at each other and shrugged their shoulders. "Why not?" they thought as they entered the dark canopy.

They didn't get far before they fell upon a huge rock face with a cave in the bottom of it.

Again, they looked at each other and said, "Let's check it out." Turning on their flashlights, they entered the cave, and after walking only a few feet, they sensed something happening to them.

Looking down at their hands and feet, they noticed a vibration, and everything was becoming a blur. Then a blinding flash of light and they were in a long swirling and twisting tunnel. Bright colors were flashing all around, and they floated freely but were turning head over heels and had no sense of gravity.

Then it was over, and they were standing on a grassy knoll near a river, but something was very wrong, and they both knew it. The grass was green, all right, but the river was orange.

Charly thought that he knew what had happened, and he explained it to Pam. "I have read about this stuff," he told her. "I think we may have stumbled on a portal to another dimension. They say there are many dimensions, and in each one, there is another you and another me doing something very different than we are doing in our normal dimension."

Pam listened.

"So, in this dimension, you may have tried to do something that you love like perhaps play the piano with hopes of being in an orchestra. But you found that you were not good at the piano, so quickly dropped that dream. But in another dimension, the same you may be a critically acclaimed pianist traveling the world and very famous." Charly finished.

Charly knew that if this was the case if they had been sucked through a portal, that they would need to remember where it was so they could return to their dimension, or they would be stuck in this world forever. He made some mental notes about the exact spot they landed and which direction they were facing when they landed. Then, they decided to explore. They would follow the orange river to see where it took them. It flowed lazily past them with a bright and luminescent orange glow. They followed it down the hill for a little way and came upon some animals. They were the size of rabbits and seemed to have the same demeanor, but their fur was bright red. They had huge bright blue eyes that looked like crystals, and they stared at the couple as they walked past.

Then, they arrived at the bottom of the hill where the river dove under a long winding road. It didn't look like a traffic road like we were accustomed to seeing but had some sort of strange metallic tracks that wove back and forth over each other.

"What sort of crazy train could fit on those tracks?" Charly asked to himself.

They crossed the unusual looking road and noticed a slight grade now going uphill again. They trudged up the hill, and when they reached the top, they both had their breath taken away for what they saw far below.

It was a massive city structure with towering pointed buildings that glowed in reds, blues, and yellow hues. It was as though the buildings themselves were radiating the light rather than being lit up by another light source as they were accustomed to in their home dimension. They saw that down at the foot of the buildings, there were waterways, and the orange river that they had followed down earlier must have been flowing down to the city.

There were also odd-looking flying crafts going in and out of the buildings at all levels. Just then, they heard a scuffling sound behind them as though somebody was walking past. They turned just in time to see a creature that was about four feet tall that had stopped and was standing and staring at them in the same way that they were now staring at it.

"Greetings, friends!" a voice said.

Charly and Pam quickly looked at each other. They had both heard the voice, and they had both been looking at the little being when they heard it, but its mouth didn't move at all.

Charly thought he knew why that was and stilled his mind. "We are visitors to your land and mean you no harm," he thought, believing that what they had heard was a telepathic communication.

"Yes, that is fine. How did you get here, and what is your name?" the voice came through again. Charly held his hands slightly out and up with the palms facing up in a gesture of friendship and took several cautious steps forwards towards the being.

"My name is Charly, and this is my wife Pam," he said, gesturing to where Pam was standing.

"Ah, good." The little being said, "we are establishing mutual communication and seeking common ground between us. I am Remicon Whaler, and it is fine to call me "Remi." It said.

Then, Charly dropped his arms and gestured to Pam to walk with him towards the being. As they got closer, they noticed that its eyes were reptilian and yellow with black vertical slits for the iris. His skin was a deep purple color and had a luminescence to it that shone the light in other colors when he moved. They saw a beautiful deep turquoise and a dark crimson that glimmered from every part of his skin. He was not wearing any clothes but looked very natural. He and no hair, and they noticed that he had large gills in the sides of his neck. Overall, he was actually quite attractive to the eyes.

"Remi, can you tell us where we are because this place is not our home. We were on vacation in Hawaii and went exploring in the jungle. We had not gone far before we were sucked into what appeared to be a wormhole or some kind of time gate. And now we are here in this beautiful place." Charly said.

"Yes, this is our home, and it is quite nice, isn't it?" Remi said. "You clearly entered by mistake, and I know how to get you back over to your dimension. You see, we here live in a closely guarded dimension, just one shift away from yours. We often use the gate you found to enter your world, but generally, there are no visitors like you ever come here. It is intriguing that you were able to do it." Remi told them.

Then Pam spoke up. "Remi, do you mind if we ask you some questions? And you, of course, can ask us as many as you like as well but we are curious. What race lives here, and are you a part of that race?" She inquired.

"Oh yes, of course, you would want to know more than just where you are, wouldn't you?" Remi mused.

"Why don't we all go to my home. It's not far from here. Would you like that?" he asked.

Remi led the way down a path we had not noticed until it came to a meadow. The path had been closely bordered by some sort of jungle plants that were about 5 to 6 feet high, and the meadow was absolutely stunning. We saw large blue trees that all had twin trunks. I don't mean that they split like our trees do, but rather came out of the ground as two separate trunks. The blue color gradually became a dark purple as it reached to heights above the meadow. The canopy was bright orange and seemed to intensify the sun's rays as they shone through it to reach us here down on the ground. And the flowers! We saw reds, blues, pinks, and white flowers everywhere. This place was much more beautiful than our home dimension, and Pam and I were amazed and impressed by it all.

"Here we are," Remi announced as we came upon what first appeared as a wall of blue wood-like substance. As I followed it up, I noticed it was actually a massive tree. The thing was so large that you could only barely determine the gradual roundness of the huge trunk. It was gargantuan. As we followed Remi towards it, a large door materialized, and we stopped before it.

Remi made an odd gesture with one of his hands, and the door opened sliding straight up. "Welcome to my home friends," Remi said as we all went inside.

Pam and I tried to cease appearing, amazed at everything when we saw the lush interior of Remi's house. I will just tell you that if the meadow was amazing, Remi's home was beyond that by many degrees. It was like walking into a massive aircraft hangar, which was furnished with Ethan Allen type furniture.

"Would you like tea?" Remi offered.

"That would be lovely," Pam responded. We both sat on a bright red soft bottom couch that must have been 25 feet long, and when we did, a recliner-like footrest seemed to come out of nowhere, and our feet were gently cradled.

"Here we go," Remi said, placing three cups of tea on the small table in front of the couch. "Please, ask your questions now." He said

Exercise

Begin by closing your eyes and imaging a peaceful world with no hurt or pain. This exrcise should be able to help be calm and happy before bed.

•This exercise has to be interactive, you are allowed to share the experience with your partner.

•The exercise should not run beyond 20 minutes

Chapter 5: The Athlete

Allison was an acrobat who thrived on the energy from her live shows with the Circus. She was a skilled young girl; she was the youngest acrobat to attempt many of her more difficult stunts. Both she and her parents

were always adamant that she took the proper safety precautions and left plenty of time for schoolwork.

She had beautiful dark skin and eyes the color of coffee, anyone who met her could tell that she was going to inherit her mother's slender face. Her loveliness was remarkable, but her talent made her who she was. Her ability to captivate an audience had won her recognition far and wide.

The whole circus treated her as a beloved daughter, which put her mother's mind at ease. Allison's parents were very protective of her and in the beginning, they were wary of her working for a circus, because of the intake of profit that was involved in running a business. The owners of the Circus were once performers themselves and dedicated to creating an environment of growth for everyone who joined their ranks.

Watching Allison as an acrobat, from the audience, was like watching a mesmerizing kaleidoscope of color-changing form from the space above. She was able to incorporate streamers into her performance, which added both color and drama to the presentation. Waves of red and green alternated out from her arms, as she hung upside down on the trapeze.

The staff had noticed her love for the bold and they worked with her to incorporate all sorts of lively music and flashy props into her show. The crowds below her cheered for the breathtaking whimsy of her act. She inspired the imaginations of thousands.

One day her mother told her that her grandparents would be visiting to see her show. She was so excited because she had a close relationship with her

whole family and could think of nothing more splendid. She made up her mind that she would create within her act, a dedication to both her mother and her grandmother. She wanted to think of something that adequately conveyed their strong nature and their importance in her own life. Her whole family was supportive of her ambitions, but her mother and grandmother had enabled her to pursue acrobatics from a young age.

She filled with a buzzing energy that night and sleep seemed to escape her. Allison was looking forward to showing her role models what they meant to her while using the skills that they had enabled her to cultivate. She remembered what use to help her when she was younger and unable to find rest. She slowed her breathing down and focused on her breath. She took deep and measured breaths in through her nose and then counted to four, then she breathed out through her mouth.

After a while, she seemed to sink through her bed, as though she were resting on a cloud. A cool and gentle wind grazed her cheek as she seemed to drift further and further down into a swirling mess of blue and purple tones hues. She remembered that purple was her grandmother's favorite color, and that's when she smelled the familiar perfume. Then the warm scent of vanilla and sugar washed over her, reminding her of a childhood spent laughing in the kitchen as her grandmother made her favorite cookies.

The environment that she had floated into was dark but not in a scary way. Allison felt what she could only describe as a feeling-echo. Love, warmth, and familiarity filled a space that seemed less like a void and more like a protective blanket. She watched as the sapphire toned wind played against the dusty pastel purple that she'd seen so much in her grandmother's clothing

while she was growing up.

That's when it struck Allison that she was in a dream. Something perhaps related to the visiting of her grandparents. She was watching her own sleeping mind's representation of her grandmother. No sooner than she realized this, she heard a soft lullaby pouring out through the darkness. A tune that held a special place in her memory, the words were fuzzy, but the emotion was all there.

She was placed gently on the ground of a forest that smelled strongly of pine, like her grandfather. He was a strong and stoic man, often silent but always present. He'd always reminded Allison of a steady and immovable evergreen tree. He watched over her and protected her. The safety of his embrace was something that comforted her, even on the worst days.

Allison sat up to observe these woods against the backdrop of berry-colored wind and sky. The space between the wild and winding trees was flecked with fireflies, dancing together under a pale golden moon. She remembered again, her childhood and the familiarity of this dreamscape. A new song was now softly ringing out through the ether, a piano like the one from her grandmother's old parties.

She stood up and began to sway back and forth to the bell-like tone of the notes. Songs from New Year's Eve with her mother's charming laughter as a background sound. For the first time since the start of the dream, Allison looked at her own attire. She was wearing a flowing yellow gown with bows and ruffles.

She decided that in the company of such a breathing and loving atmosphere, she would try some stunts. Allison had never had a lucid dream before and was eager to test out her skills. She found a path through the trees and began running to prepare for a flip.

As she turned over and over in the cool night air, she realized that she had grown brilliant wings. They were decorated like a Monarch butterfly, with black outlining pockets of lava red and orange. Her own wings were in stark contrast to the cool colors that were still swirling around her.

She decided to fly around and see what wonders she might find. She was passing the fireflies as she made her ascension. Both her mother and her grandmother had always loved Monarchs. They had always kept certain plants around that encouraged visits from butterflies. She remembered, noticing that she looked like a soaring tapestry of flames.

She passed over a beautiful body of water with quite an unusual pink glow, and she could not help but think of a sunset's reflection on a mountain lake. This was something else that she had locked away in a deep part of her brain, something that could only be a memory.

The young girl soared above the piney trees, flipping, and twirling in the air. She was having so much fun; taking full advantage of the freedom offered by the night sky. She took several deep breaths, inhaling the perfumed air. Allison was taken by the beauty of distant twinkling stars.

She was flying through the night air at such a speed, that she didn't even notice the chorus of other flying creatures that had joined her in flight. Birds,

bats, and butterflies all began flying right alongside the young girl as she ventured further and further out.

Allison watched as the landscape below her changed from trees to water, and then back again. The feeling of being free in the air was a good part of the reason that she had always dreamed of being an acrobat. To her, the air was synonymous with happiness.

This dreamscape went on forever and soon Allison found herself watching the dark sky, fade into a sunrise peppered with lovely cotton candy pink clouds. She knew that she was dreaming and therefore hoped that all these cotton clouds would actually taste of candy.

She flew toward the clouds with a determination to taste them. The moment she reached her destination, she awoke to her mother's voice in her ear. She had slept through the entire night while preoccupied with her dream symphony.
Allison had some many good ideas now and used them to map out her next show. She would include so many of these unconscious memories in order to honor the strong women in her family. She had absolutely fallen in love with the idea of including some sort of butterfly imagery in her act.

The young girl had her work cut out for her, as she had never designed everything about her act before. There was always someone older and more knowledgeable there to advise her decisions. She was going to endeavor to have full creative control over this one.

Allison told management about her request and they were understandably hesitant to allow someone so young to plan out their act. In the end, they agreed with the stipulation that she run everything by them before opening night and include all of the proper safety precautions.

Allison put together a magnificent performance that entailed her dressing as a butterfly and unfurling her wings while in the air. The audience was cheered for her daring stunts and in the conclusion of her show, she received a standing ovation for her act. Her ideas were a hit.

That night when she returned to the safety of her own home, both her mother and her grandmother commended her bravery. She told them that their influence in her life was the driving force in her show, and they were both touched. Her mom began to cry tears of joy in response to this sentiment. Her

grandmother was smiling to herself.
Allison was the talk of the circus when she returned. Every staff member was in awe of the beauty and grace that she showcased as an acrobat. Allison had managed to capture the imaginations of even her peers.

Chapter 6: Holiday on the Island

"Can we swim wif the dolphins 'gain, Mommy?"

"Finish brushing your teeth first!" Jenny called into the bathroom.

The silly child poked her head out of the bathroom, toothbrush in hand, lips covered in toothpaste.

"Okie, Mom!" Flecks of toothpaste flew as she said it, and then grinned with foamy teeth.

Kirsty came out wiping her mouth with the back of her long sleeve and hopped into the bed as Jenny pulled back the covers.

"I really like the dolphins, Mom. They know how to have fun!"

"They do." Jenny nodded. "But there are all kinds of dreams to explore, you know. There is an entire world full of them out there. All kinds of perspectives you never imagined."

"What does 'perspective' mean, Mommy?"

Jenny tapped a finger to her lips.

"It's...it's a way you view the world. Do you know how you got to see the forest dreaming from the fox's view? That's a new perspective."

"Oh, okay! So what kind of per-spec-tive are we going to see tonight?"

Jenny opened the book, it is cover crackling. She flipped through the pages until she came to the next chapter.

"Oh, yes. This is a special one."

She turned the book so that Kirsty could properly see the picture.

It depicted a tropical island, thick with palm trees and ferns, and fallen coconuts on the beach forming a pattern that looked like the numeral "3."

Above it, in the swaying branches and green canopy, peeked all sorts of brightly colored birds.

Their many calls mingled with the sound of the lapping waves to create a light and hopeful background.

The scent of salt and the pungent fragrance of tropical plants drifted from the pages.

"Now, sweetie, let me show you what the dolphins were so keen to get to explore, but from a different perspective...."

* * *

Jaina woke up on a beach, but not the beach she had left.

Now instead of a sandy path back to the city, she found herself on a tropical island.

Coconuts littered the sand at her feet.

Bright red and spiky fruits hung in some of the trees.

A warm tropical wind blew past, stirring the leaves with a whispering rustle and billowing her hair.

Jaina smiled as she breathed it in. The air smelled so fresh, a lingering tang on her tongue.

She turned toward the nearby jungle.

A small bird with green feathers and a shiny blue around its head hopped down from one of the branches.

"Welcome!" it chirped. "This is my home. Do you like it?"

Jaina nodded enthusiastically.

"It's wonderful. So warm and cozy and peaceful. How do you ever stay awake here? I think I would spend my day napping if I lived in such a nice place!"

"Oh, but you don't know what else there is to see!" said Bird.

"You would have no time for napping all day if you could see the beauty of this place!"

"Could I? Could you show me?" Jaina looked hopeful, her eyes big and bright.

The bird could not resist her plea.

"Yes, I will show you. Come with me and see what only one on the wing can see! Then you tell me if you would spend all day napping."

"Deal!"

Jaina held out her arm, and Bird alighted upon it, tilting its head back and forth to stare at her with each eye.

"And...let the wind takes us!"

Then it flew off again, and Jaina found that she was looking at the beach from high above.

She was like Bird, winging her way through warm blue skies to appreciate the jungle and the ocean from on high.

She circled higher and higher, and the whole island became a green-carpeted seed below her.

Up until this high in the sky, only the winds kept her company, singing of the distant waves, of the past and the future.

"Here we go!" Bird dove down, tucking her wings, as the green jungle rushed up to meet her.

She spread her wings and arced smoothly into level flight, circling the treetops.

Below her, she saw the coconuts sitting in the trees, humming softly in the breeze.

Harsh voices rose up to meet her: monkeys leaping from branch to branch, picking the fruits and eating them with lyrical delight.

They looked up at Bird as she flew past and waved their hands in envy.

Into the canopy, she plunged.

Green fan-shaped leaves fluttered in the wind as she flew past.

Other birds, some of them yellow with black beaks, and some of the dark blue with yellow beaks, and still others red with white markings sang loudly, all competing voices.

They looked up as she flew past. Some rose into the air with a flutter of feathers, but they could not keep up with her speed.

She wove through corridors of green and tan, leaves and branches adorned with fruits or coconuts, nimbly winging around tree trunks, dodging hanging vines, and great big spiderwebs glistening with morning dew like living chandeliers.

The chorus of chirps and hooting cries followed her as she raced through a blur of the jungle.

Then she was free and flew out over the beach, above the water.

Fish leaped and swam in the cerulean waves, all aglow from the sunshine warming the world.

Dolphins cavorted off the shore, leaping high from white-capped waves to glisten in the sun and crash back down again.

Bird Jaina watched the shadows darting about beneath the surface, and then she turned back to the island.
Flocks of seabirds circled on the shores, diving down to peck at some meal washed ashore.

"Food! Food! Food!" their cries said.

The bird had more on her mind than simply eating.

She circled the island, white sand streaming by beneath her, the lush jungle rotating slowly in her eyes.

Slender fingers of sunlight crept through the canopy and golden dust swirled in their grasp.

Little lizards and dark beetles crawled up the trunks, racing to the top to reach the sunlight. Their voices rose ever higher in competition.

The bird let out a warbling song to drown them out. Her voice echoed in the jungle as she spiraled ever higher, eventually reaching high above the island once more.

"This is an amazing view!" said Jaina.

"Yes, it is." Bird tucked her wings and dove once more.

"But sometimes you need to see from a bird's eye view up close!"

Down she flew into the jungle canopy, landing upon a high branch.

The wind caressed her feathers as she preened her wing, and then looked down on the world unfolding below her.

In the thick undergrowth, many creatures crawled, each with a voice of its own.

A furry anteater hummed its slow, ponderous song as it wandered lazily through the brush, long tongue flicking out of its long face.

The anteater stopped and looked up at Bird as she sang down to it.

"Good…morning…" said the anteater, it is every word drawn out and rolling.

"It is a good morning!" said Bird. "But there are no ants up here, my friend."

"That's…okay." The anteater plodded along on its search.

A soft croak drew her attention, followed by another, and another.

Small frogs with very vibrant coloring hopped up the tree trunk.

Bird knew better than to test them: they were beautiful but dangerous if you were careless, much like the sweetest of dreams.

One of the frogs, neon green with red sides, leaped from the tree as a wind sighed through the palm fronds.

The frog spread into wings of luminous glass, a butterfly with glowing blue and black patterns on its wings.

As Bird and Jaina watched the butterfly shattered into a hundred tiny slivers of blue light, and each grew wings, a sudden swarm of sky-blue butterflies shining in the shaded forest canopy.

Laughing, Bird flew down to join them, and suddenly found herself caught within a cloud of swirling blue.

They spiraled with the wind, down nearly to the ground and then back up into the branches, pushing through the leaves and emerging into the sunlight beyond.

As the butterflies flew, a symphony of fluttering notes filled the air.

The bird stopped flapping her wings and for a moment just drifted up on the music of the island itself: the rush of wings, wind, and waves, all joining together to create a warm sound.

The frond-leaves were as wings, emerald feathers joining her in flight.

Whole flocks rose out of the green to take to the sky with her, and they soared so high even the wind envied them.

Blue skies opened up before them, and to Jaina's delight, she found they soared higher still.

Into kingdoms of cloud they flew, where mountains of mist and moisture rolled past, and visions of the ancient world rose up and fell away in mere moments.

Clouds became like islands in the sky, floating upside down in an airy ocean.

The wind rolled through it all like oceanic currents, some warm and lazy, some cool and swift.

The flock changed again, leaves borne upon the wind, now clad in white cloud-feathers, wreathed in a scent of rain.

Thunder rolled and the islands gave way to a downpour, cascading from the clouds as waterfalls.

The flock dove into the rain, becoming like fish of sea green, fins like wings, but the music never changed.

The song of the island: that of sea and sky, where the voices of the waves and the dreams of the wind combined.

Therefore, down they fell, back into the water, bursting through the surface and emerging from a geyser of bubbles in yet another world.

There the deep blue embraced them, warm and salty, and they sank into its liquid softness. Currents enveloped them.

Colorful ocean fish darted back and forth amid the reefs that surrounded the island, and the flock changed yet again, becoming like them, bright and quick, yet trailing seaweed from their tails.

Longer and longer, the trails grew, as they flew through the water around the island, binding it in green.

The land became green beneath them, and the clouds of fish were as clouds in the sky, glimpsed through the shimmering surface above them.

Green seaweed beds settled onto coral and melted together into trees with palm leaves and the rocks that once adorned the reef hung from the trees like coconuts.

Sun shone through the surface, upon which the shadows of swaying trees danced.

She landed beside a pool in the center of it all that slowly filled up with clear gleaming water.

The bird looked into the pool and Jaina was there beside her, staring at their reflections.

She sat back and laughed. "That was amazing!

I never knew the island was so perfectly poised between the two worlds."

"Three," said Bird cheerily.

"Earth, sea, and sky. This little island offers them all for those who want them. Even for one who has hopped and flown every single inch of this island. Do you see now why I never tire of it? To nap here would be divine, but if this whole place is like a dream come to life, would you need to?"

Jaina sat back on her hands. The warm tropical air stirred her hair and tasted faintly of salt.

She smiled.

"I think it would be hard to tell the difference. This entire place is perfect. As you said, it's got something for everyone."

A coconut fell and rolled down a little sandy hill, bumping lightly into her knee.

Jaina picked it up and found that it already had a straw in it, drawn from the little reeds that surrounded the pool.

She sipped at the sweet coconut milk, the taste rolling over her tongue like the white clouds through which they had flown.

Jaina lay back on a bed of soft, fragrant tropical flowers.

Closing her eyes and just relishing the tastes of the island, Jaina did not even notice the coconut slip from her fingers.

The birds continued their endless cries around her, and the wind continued to caress the waves.

Jaina fell into dreams that were little different from the waking beauty that was the island life.

Bioluminescence

In the waters of the darkened deep
A world of magical creatures swim and creep
Jellyfish undulating, glowing blue, purple, or green
Unnamed creatures never before are seen
Creatures of living light, so impossible to believe
A thought one would never conceive
Brilliant underwater light show,
A million, swimming fish all aglow
Glowing plants too, swaying with the ocean waves
Along the sea bottom and lighting up underwater caves
The magic of this place, as the sea creatures float and shimmer
A haven of peace for a weary soul; a dreamtime swimmer

Dreams and Sea Glass

Once, alone I went to the shore
Looking for sea glass but found something more
There were the land meets the sea
I was found by a kindred soul, and he spoke to me
He said "Hello" and we talked for a while
Of our dreams and places, we had been, and then we shared a smile
One thing neither of us could possibly know
Was how in time this friendship would grow
Little by little their dreams our dreams we would share
And slowly, day by day we started to care
In time, he became a best friend none could surpass
Walking along the shore, sharing dreams and sea glass

Mirror

I wish I had a mirror to reflect
To show you yourself, in circumspect
That you could truly see the soul inside,
And look at yourself with pride
I want you to know, how beautiful you are
To see that you can do so much; go so far
To know the gentleness, you possess
And to see, that you can be a success
I wish I had that mirror to show
So, you could see and you could know
That you are amazing, talented, and smart
That you have a poet's soul and a golden heart

The Wind

The wind kisses my cheeks and it blows by
It lingers for a moment, then leaves; no one knows why
The wind whispers its secrets to the trees
Then blows away in a playful breeze
Leaves dance, and whirlwinds blow
The wind, delighting us with her show
A whimsical elemental friend
Ever changing, ever-present. The Wind.

Chapter 7: The Beautiful Summer

The summer was as gorgeous as any Jenny had known.

Days of running through the sprinklers, and going out to the lake, and having picnics in the local park.

Roasting marshmallows in the fire pit out in the backyard, making s' mores, and enjoying family get-togethers around the barbecue.

The weather was warm but cold lemonade and shade under the trees helped to keep everyone cool.

Jenny worked hard and brought about many changes: remodeling the home, taking on a new role at work, helping her daughter recover from her very first exciting school year.

Tonight, Jenny sat with Kirsty out by the fire pit in the fading evening light.

The others had gone inside, but she wanted to spend the night with her daughter and enjoy one of the last nights of summer.

The smell of wood smoke drifted on the air. Gentle pops and crackles accompanied the embers that floated up in the air, glimmered, and went out.

One of Jenny's favorite things in the whole world was to sit next to a fire and enjoy the warmth and flickering glow, and the sound, the smell, all of it. She loved it, and now she had passed that down to her daughter, as well.

The steady sound of crickets and the occasional hoot of a night bird made a relaxing chorus to lull their heavy eyelids ever down further.

"I want a story, Mom," said Kirsty, yawning heavily in her chair. Then she hugged the blanket she had brought outside even closer around her.

Her head leaned back, but she was not ready yet. Jenny had brought out a sleeping bag because sometimes they liked to sleep out under the stars, on perfect nights like tonight.

Kirsty got out of her chair, went over to the sleeping bag, and slid into it, the fabric swishing loudly as she snuggled in.

Jenny moved her chair over near the sleeping bag.

"I thought you might, honey, so I came prepared!"

Jenny lifted the book she had had sitting beside the chair: their favorite storybook.

"How are you going to read in the dark, Mommy?"

The flickering firelight did not offer much steady light for reading, but Jenny only smiled.

Jaina ran barefoot through the dandelion fields.

Soft grass and cold, moist dandelions comforted her feet as she ran, springing up again as she passed through.

Other flowers stood amid the dandelions but she loved them all equally. There were white flowers and pink and blue ones, all set against the deepest green grass, and the dandelions shone like droplets fallen from the sun on high.

The smell was so divine! Aromatic grass, wild and thick, met with the fragrances of sweet nectar.

Breathing it in was like feeling the soft petals gently caressing her face. Jaina could never get tired of it.

She knelt down and scooped a fuzzy white dandelion out of the earth. Holding it aloft, some of the seeds began to blow away on the wind.

Jaina watched them float, and she laughed because that was exactly what she wanted to wish for.

"I wish I could fly as you do, and see what you see!"

Then she pursed her lips and blew, scattering all but one seed from the dandelion head.

Countless flowers waved in the breeze, each a little point of light, like a star in a deep emerald sky. About them wove beautiful music, thousands upon thousands of voices raised up together in song.

The wind whooshed and the dandelion seed soared as the ground fell away in rolling hills. She lifted higher into the sky, where winds flowed like river currents in an invisible ocean.

The sky darkened. Something passed by overhead, giving out a proud cry.

It was an eagle, soaring with its feathers in the sun. Jaina beamed as she looked up at it.

She had always loved birds, admired their freedom in flight, and now she has to experience the same thing.

The dandelion seed caught an updraft and higher she went still, hot on the tail of the mighty eagle.

Floating beside it, she laughed, and tears streamed from her face, in sheer joy.

This was something she had always wanted, and now her wish had come true!

Trees rose like spires from the land, each holding an entire world in their branches.

The eagle saw all: the scurrying squirrels and the nesting birds, the hares and the deer, the fish gleaming in the far-away streams winding about the feet of the trees.

Here, this place was alive with the fullness of the summer, an inexhaustible flame of vitality.

Beyond the green and growing things, the eagle saw the spirits of land and sky, which frolicked as happily as a bird on the wing.

They were tiny like Jaina, or big like the eagle, sometimes both at once. Their lives mirrored that of the land itself.

Where they trod, life bloomed, and where life bloomed, they gravitated, forever finding meaning in the growth of the smallest seed, or the tranquility of the tallest tree.

Jaina realized that even during the day, when most were wide-awake and stretching out beneath the sun, the world dreamed, and she floated through its dreams at once an observer and a fellow traveler.

She breathed in deeply as the wind rushed across her face, granting her a sense of freedom she had never know before.

Here, sailing upon the sky itself, she knew what the golden days of late summer meant to all that lived within them.

She could feel the vibrant pulse of the world hot in her veins. It gave her such a sense of purpose, an invigoration that nothing else could match.

"You must not forget this feeling," said the eagle.

"This is life, my friend. Life at its purest. Enjoying sun, star, and moon. Breathing in the wind. Flying freely. You could weigh as much as a tree and still not burden me, for I am free. Here you are free, too."

A rocky outcropping stood tall over the bank of a wide blue lake below.

The eagle dipped his head. "Farewell, friend! Return whenever it pleases you!"

Jaina dove from the eagle's head turned and waved goodbye to him as she fell.

She spread her arms and let the wind slip through her fingers, cool and soft.

The lake grew as she fell toward it, but she was not afraid. Like a drop of rain, she broke the surface and plunged into another world.

The lake welcomed her as it welcomed the sunlight, which cast rays that soon became swirling mist within the waves.

And in the water's cold, refreshing embrace she saw more travelers. Big, silvery fish, their eyes bigger than her sprite-sized body, swam past, lazily enjoying the warm waters.

Jaina found that she could move through the water as freely as the eagle had the air, and she glided over to a bed of kelp that grew outward like a swaying forest.

A soft song like a hum rose from the kelp, celebrating its perspective: a green plant that enjoyed both water and sun in equal measure.

Jaina reached out and touched one of the leafy stalks and for a moment saw what the kelp saw: an entire kingdom stretching out across the bottom of the lake, and a sky ever shimmering at the surface.

Fish hid within its leafy mass. Crawdads crawled across the silt within its reach. Frogs and tadpoles danced to its endless tune. Ducks in the water sent ripples ringing like notes across the wave-sky above.

Pieces of driftwood floated by and some of the kelp would seize onto it, pulled free to drift with the wood.

The kelp saw all these lives bound together by the water and the growing earth and the sweet air above. Its perspective was truly blessed, to know so much of the lake's grand symphony.

Jaina swam back to the surface, buoyed by the haze of sunlight filtering down through the water.

She surfaced, listening to the plink and splash of the water.

Jaina lay back and closed her eyes, floating like a flower petal and simply enjoying the relaxing sounds.

She slept, or perhaps sleeping was the same as waking here, where dream and reality were one.

When she opened her eyes, no time had passed at all. The sun was still high in the sky above the lake, and a warmth rippled across the water.

Her breathing coincided with the rise and fall of the gentle waves. In, the water rose, lifting her toward the sky. Out, the water sank, and she felt cradled in a cool liquid bed.

In. Out. A year could have rolled past and she was so calm she would have never noticed it.

Presently a deep hum beat the air. Jaina opened her eyes.

A dragonfly hovered over the lake surface nearby, landing on a small piece of driftwood.

To the rest of the world, it was only a few inches long, but to Jaina the traveler, it looked to be closer in size to an actual dragon!

"Hello!" she called, waving. The dragonfly turned its head to her and its wings buzzed.

"Hello. Fine day, is it not?"

"Yes, it is!" Jaina clapped, incredibly amused that the dragonfly had answered her. "I have never enjoyed the lake so much."

The dragonfly buzzed in agreement. "Oh yes. The sun is pleasant and the water is refreshing. But I must be going. Will you need a lift?"

Jaina's eyes lit up.

Jaina looked down at the lake slowly strolling past beneath her, an amazing view of its shimmering surface from high up.

Never before had she had such a perfect wish granted?

A white cloud descended to fly next to her—no, not a cloud, the dandelion seed.

The very same one, she was sure of it.

"Thank you!" she called to the dragonfly before she let go and took hold of the floating seed again.

"May the winds bear you to wherever your heart desires!" called the dragonfly, and then he flew back down toward the lakeshore.

But Jaina floated upward and upward, the lake shrinking beneath her.

Soon she plunged into the clouds, rolling white mountains of mist and magic.

Jaina saw shapes therein: faces, animals, trees, castles. She saw glistening streams of water spiraling through the clouds like the dreams of rain. Cool moisture kissed her skin, warmed again by the sun when they emerged into the open blue air.

Jaina had never tasted such pure, sweet air, tinged with the scent of a fresh-fallen rain.

When the sunbeams hit the clouds just the right way they glittered like a field of stars.

Then one of the clouds would break and a torrent of rain fell, shining colors like stained glass as it poured down to the earth. Each raindrop was a different note and created the perfect symphony of sun and sky as she listened.

The dandelion seed passed through a wisp of cloud and Jaina, lulled nearly to sleep, let go.

She waved. "Farewell! Thank you for letting me fly with you!"

The seed floated slowly away, vanishing into the clouds, where its own dreams had always taken it.

Jaina lay back in a bed of pure softness, white like snow, warm like a lake in the sun, and clear as the air after a cleansing rainstorm. She spread her arms wide and closed her eyes.

A soft sound like the sighing of wind mingled with the gentle slosh of lake water filled all her mind.

Then she grew content, more so than she had ever known, freed as the wind and water, birds and clouds, from the burdens of her daily stresses.

Jaina slept in a sea of clouds and the smile never left her lips.

Chapter 8: The Lovely Fish

A long time ago, deep down the sea, there lived a young angelfish with his family. His family and friends knew the angelfish by the name of Tobi. Isaacused to play with his brother, Kish, and many of his friends.

Life at sea was fun, and the young fishes used to spend most of their time playing. One of their favorite games was deep-diving. They would swim to great depths, almost near the surface, and then they would race back home at high speed, always competing against each other. Kish was an excellent racer, always out-competing his peers.

"You, crab, you are very old. You cannot compete with a champion like me," Kish would always say, thumping his chest at anyone giving him any attention.

Although Isaacwas not that good at racing as his brother, he was very gifted in singing. He had the most melodious voice in the neighborhood. Whenever he was alone, he would be heard singing some of his favorite songs. He was always found singing even while carrying out the assigned duties at home. He had composed a song for almost every activity. There was a song for scrapping the floor, a song for tending the flower, one for doing the dishes, and another for vacuuming or doing the laundry. His mother had noticed that whenever her favorite son was singing, he was always happy. On the other hand, his father was a little concerned that all the singing might interfere with his son's academic career. He desperately wanted Isaacto be a doctor, just like the king whale's famous son.

"I wonder what will become of Tobi's singing. Will he want to change his career to music instead of medicine?" he often mused loudly to himself or to

whoever was around him.

"My husband, let the young man be. He is only a young child. Besides, music is also an excellent career," Tobi's mother always came to his defense.

"Alright, dear. As long as it does not interfere with his career, let us support him."

"Thank you, my husband. I always knew I married a very reasonable man!"

And so it happened during Tobi's eighth birthday. His parents surprised him with a full set of musical instruments. He couldn't believe his eyes when he arrived home from the playground and found all the beautiful music instruments neatly arranged in his room. There was a guitar, piano, keyboard, violin, flute, and saxophone. He was so excited. He kept running his delicate fingers on the instruments.

"Thank you so much, mom and dad. This is the best birthday gift ever," he excitedly told his parents.

"Welcome, son," they replied.

"You are the best parents ever." He said, hugging them in a tight embrace. Then he rushed out, his friends and the whole world had to know of his newest, fanciest possessions.

The following days, the whole neighborhood was filled with melodious music coming from Tobi's house. The community appreciated Tobi's unique

gift, and soon, he started becoming a famous musician. He started getting invites to grace special events like birthdays and wedding ceremonies. He was a forthcoming young musician.

However, Isaachad a problem unknown to many. He had two challenges. The first was he had not mastered well how to play to the saxophone. And the second was he had difficulty performing before a large crowd. Wherever he was on stage, he found the many pairs of eyes very intimNylating. He had tried mastering his challenge with no success. Finally, he decided to seek help on how to overcome his problem. He decided to ask his brother's opinion first.

"Bro, I have something to tell you. It is a problem that has been disturbing me for a while now," he started. They were sitting at the terrace beside their house. This was one of their favorite places to hang out.

"You can always tell me anything. Go ahead, champion," said his brother.

"I have two problems. One, I can't play this thing quite well. I have tried, but it is almost getting beyond me!" he said, pointing at the saxophone that he was carrying.

"Well, if you have tried hard enough with no results, perhaps you can get some training. I suggest you see Master, the Frog. He is the best music teacher around," his brother replied expertly.

"Thanks a lot, brother; I knew I could rely on you! Isaacsaid excitedly. Although he had known Master all his life, he had never thought of approaching him for help.

"No worries. What are brothers for? What is your second problem? You mentioned you had two problems."

"Well, it is not a challenge per see, but it is still a problem. I have a problem with the crowd."

"The crowd! How, brother? The crowd loves you. You should see how they go wild whenever you hit the stage," Kish exclaimed excitedly.

"I don't know. I find myself freezing at the sight of a big crowd."

"Well, maybe you'll get advice on how to overcome your challenge once you see Mr. Frog."

So the following morning, Isaacwas the first to knock at Master Frog's house. "Come in, young man. What can I do for you?" asked Master Frog as he welcomed him warmly. He was used to receiving young kids who were seeking his help in building a successful music career. Whenever he could, he always helps such promising talents.

Isaacpromptly explained his problem to Master Frog, who listened attentively. He was sitting in his sizeable imposing desk next to the large piano.

"I will help you with your problems, Tobi, but let's start with the saxophone first," he told Tobi.

The following day, they dedicated a lot of their time learning how to play the saxophone. Isaacwas a swift learner, and Master Frog was impressed with his talent. He decided to enroll Isaacin the International Music Competition, which was to take place in the next few coming months.

But Master Frog knew that for Isaacto compete well, he had to get rid of his stage fright problem. He wondered how best to help the young champion. Then an idea struck him. Smiling to himself, he picked up the phone and made a call to Tobi's house.

"Hello, how can I help you?" It was Tobi's mother who was on the other end of the phone.

"It's Master Frog here. Is Isaacin? I would appreciate it if you would hand the phone to him," Master Frog told Tobi's mother.

"Wait a moment," she replied, and Master Frog could hear Tobi's mother shouting for him to come down and receive the call. Then in a few more minutes, Isaacwas on the other end of the phone.

"Hello, Master, it is an honor to hear your voice. I wasn't expecting your call at all," he said, surprised at what might have made Master call him at such an hour.

"Well, Tobi, it is about your problem. The stage fright problem, you remember? I think I got a perfect solution for it. Please be at my place very early tomorrow morning," Mater Frog instructed him through the phone.

"Thank you so much, Master. I will be at your place very early," Isaacsaid excitedly.

He knew how vital confidence was, especially in winning a major competition like the international music competition. He hoped to overcome his problem quickly and in time for the upcoming competition.

The following morning, Isaacwent to Mr. Frog's house. He found him cooking some delicious breakfast. They sat down to eat breakfast, and then Master started talking.

"Tobi, there is an easy way to overcome your stage, fright," Mr. Frog began. "What is it? I am willing to learn it all, sir," said Isaaceagerly.
"It is straightforward, Tobi. Wherever you feel frightened, take a deep breath."

"Deep breaths?" asked Isaacin disbelief.

"Yes, deep breaths, more than three times. To steady your nerves," Master Frog replied.

"Will it really work?" asked Isaacin disbelief.

"Well, why don't we find out? On the count of three, close your eyes and take three deep breaths," Master instructed.

Isaacclosed his eyes, and following the instructions of Mr. frog, he took three deep breaths. He repeated the exercise over and over again. And sure enough, he found his confidence level starting to rise.

"Let us do it together," Mr. Frog encouraged him," One—" they inhaled deeply, then released the breath

"Two," they repeated. The more they did the exercise, the more Isaac felt more confident about himself. He vowed to implement the instructions every day. Mr. Frog had insisted that for Isaac to succeed, he had to make practice as part of his daily routine. Sure enough, in the subsequent days, Isaac concentrated on the exercises even during his local performance. And the best part of it was that it was working for him.

Finally, the big day of the competition arrived. Tobi, together with his parents and brother, Kish, traveled to the next kingdom to attend the contest. Mr. Frog, too, was in attendance. He had promised to participate in giving Isaac the necessary support.

There were so many participants and spectators. It was a significant event that attracted a big pool of participants. It was apparent the competition was going to be very stiff. One by one, the participants were called on the stage. And they outdid themselves in giving their best performances. Finally, it was Tobi's turn to be on stage. To say that he wasn't frightened was a lie. Once he stood on the podium and surveyed the arena, he almost fainted. There were far too many eyes staring up at him. But then he remembered Mr. Frog's advice. He steadied himself up and inhaled deeply three times. Then he repeated the exercise, and soon, he calms down enough, and his confidence

level rose. Then he picked his saxophone and gave the most electrifying performance that got; the whole crowd was on their feet. It was the best performance of the event.

Finally, when the judges announced the winners of the competition, Tobi's name was on top of the list. His parents were so excited, so was his brother, Kish, and his mentor, Mr. Frog. Isaac went on to win major competitions across the sea world. He established his career as the best musician.

Chapter 9: The Camping Excursion

The last night of their camping excursion dawned and Jenny sat with her daughters out in the cool night air.

She breathed deeply. The scent of recent rain was sweet.

Nearby, the lake waves reflected the last rays of the setting sun into a golden sheen.

Everything felt washed clean and refreshed. Evergreen trees towered over the campsites, giving off the tangy aroma of pine sap.

A few birds still hooted and chirped in the trees, but one by one, they were dropping off into silence, leaving the crackling and popping fire to mingle with the soft lake sounds.

Jenny sat in a camping chair by the fire, holding her youngest to her chest. Kirsty sat in the chair beside her, hugging a blanket around herself. The orange firelight danced upon their features.

Stars appeared in the sky overhead, white gems set upon a blue tapestry.

Jenny craned her head back to look up at them, and Kirsty followed suit.

Some stars shone brighter than others did, some were steady, and some flickered rapidly. The view was enchanting. At last Kirsty spoke.

"Mommy, do you ever wonder what's out there?"

"All the time, sweetie. I used to dream of it quite a lot. I wanted to be an astronaut when I was your age. I still think it'd be amazing to go out there and explore someday."

"I wanna be an astronaut, Mommy! Could I?"

"Baby, you know we've always told you to just follow your dreams. If you want to be an astronaut and see the stars or an astrophysicist and see what makes them work, you should do that."

"But what if I want to see what the stars dream, Mom? Do you think the stars and planets dream like that?"

Jenny smiled. "Well, then I suppose you'd be an artist, hon. Poets, painters, writers, performers, they've all been inspired at times by the view from down here. I used to paint some when I was a kid, too. I used to know the trick to making the paintings really come to life!"

"Aww, I'll bet you could still do it, Mommy! Just like your book!"

At that, Jenny grinned knowingly. "You mean this book, dear? This one right here?" She lifted the heavy book and opened it to one of the last chapters.

"You asked what it was like to become a dreamer of the stars. Well, let me show you a small piece of that place. It's pretty amazing...."

The picture that graced the page was a galaxy spinning in a milky torrent of stars.

Beyond it, one could see vast nebulas and cosmic pathways leading to the ineffable mysteries of the universe.

But the stars shone so brightly that for a moment before Jenny turned the page, night turned to day within the endless night of space itself.

Kirsty gasped, and then her mother turned the page....

* * *

Jaina leaned her head against the window as the miles rolled past.

Back through the desert, where things were open and quiet, back home to the city.

She would be glad to be home but it was hard to leave such beauty behind.

As she looked up, she saw one particular star twinkle ever brighter.

It seemed to beckon her gaze and her flight of fancy. She wondered at its impossibly long life and its incalculable distance from her.

What had it seen in all its many years, way out there in space?

Jaina imagined that even stars had dreams, or maybe the entire universe itself was like a dream to them. After all, their perspective was so different from hers down on Earth.

As her eyelids began to close, lulled by the gentle hum of the moving car, she wondered just what it was like to look down from such a height....

When Jaina opened her eyes, she found that she was floating alone in the dark. No, not in the dark. A light shone in her face.

It took her eyes a moment to adjust.

She realized that she was looking up at the half-shadowed face of the moon, but it was so close! It filled nearly her whole field of vision.

She could almost reach out and touch it.

Jaina turned and saw below her the Earth in all its glory: blue and green, white swirling clouds forming pleasant shapes she recognized as birds, mice, flowers, and more.

Jaina just floated, breathlessly awed by the sight.

She had never realized how magnificent the world was, so vast in its infinite varieties and mysteries.

What a place to call home!

From here, she could even hear its song, a grand symphony formed by the smallest organism to the largest mountain in unison. Nothing could compare.

Another song called to her.

It was the Moon, a sweet note of admiration for the Earth that was its home as well. Jaina floated toward the moon and landed upon its surface.

It spoke to her in a voice that was both young and old, lilting and yet soothing. "Hello, little one. You travel far tonight. It pleases me that you can hear me sing to my greatest love."

Jaina beamed proudly. "Yes, I can! I have never heard the Moon like this before. Or the Earth. I am very happy to have gotten a chance to experience it. This is what it's like for you all the time?"

The Moon glowed happily. "The notes change depending on where I am, which is why I circle the whole world. I want to hear everything and everyone."

"Of course!" Jaina sprang lightly up, floating far above the surface of the moon. "I do, too. It is why I came out this far tonight. I really want to see what it's like outside of what I know."

"Then you will need to go very far tonight, little one! Let my gravity help you along, and remember to say goodnight when you come this way again." And the Moon exerted her gravity, propelling Jaina in a wide arc around her white surface.

Jaina laughed and cheered, feeling as though she was caught up in a sudden gust out in a place where no air existed. She waved farewell to the Moon as she sailed away.

A huge red planet greeted her with a bombastic song, like an entire orchestra of crashing cymbals and bellowing tubas.

Vast mountains and deep valleys scrawled across its surface gave the impression of a starkly rising and falling melody.

Craters pocked the surface, and in each one danced lights of peculiar color, always in some pattern.

Waves and snowflake-like formations, rippling circles, and stranger shapes appeared.
The dreams of Mars itself met with those of the people on Earth looking outward at the red planet, and the result was an aurora-like luminescence that blanketed the red planet. Thrilled, Jaina flew onward.

Far ahead, asteroids lay across her field of vision like dark flowers upon a starry black lawn.

Jaina swam freely through the open space to them, growing larger with each passing second.

There were small asteroids and medium-sized ones, and ones so huge they were like buildings floating in nothingness.

Some spun according to their own inertia, some floated motionlessly, and still, others turned this way and that.

Jaina landed upon one and found that she was not alone.

Little sprites danced merrily between pieces of asteroids, disappearing into one of the many holes in their porous surfaces only to emerge again with a cackle and a flash.

Jaina tried to follow them but they were too swift for her, ever urging her on with their laughter and frolicking.

Jaina leaped after one and it vanished in a puff, but she sailed into the tunnel into the asteroid.

Metals or gleaming crystals sparkled as she flew through a tunnel that rang with voices of fairies and capricious spirits of space and time.

Light-filled the tunnel like a sudden sun, but when she reached the other side, she found that she had only come back to the beginning.
The laughter of the fairies greeted her from within the tunnel.

Jaina laughed in turn. Their games were not malicious, just tricky.

"Okay, keep your secrets! I think I'm too big to fit, anyway!"

"Size is very relative here," said one of the spirits, appearing like a miniature ghostly star wreathed in cosmic dust.

In one moment, it was small as a baseball, and when Jaina blinked for that instant, the spirit seemed inconceivably vast as the Sun.

"In the dreams of the universe, 'big' or 'small' is meaningless. You are as important as the biggest asteroid, the smallest sun. The galaxy could not exist without you, and you could not exist without the galaxy!"

Jaina's eyes grew wide. "Oooh, I think I don't quite understand, but I want to!"

"Then journey further. All that is beckons you."

Jaina thanked the spirit and she drifted further still, past the asteroid belt.

As soon as she crossed that border, the music of the cosmos changed. It became loftier, more harmonic, and resonant in a way that reached into her deepest thoughts.

She closed her eyes and listened, content to be merely a part of the music of the spheres for a moment, an eternity.

When she opened her eyes again, she found that she had drifted near to a truly giant planet, a great swirling mass of browns and reds and cream colors, with a swirling eye roving this way and that.

Presently it turned to her, and she found that the world was speaking to her. Its voice was slow and sonorous, and it sounded a lot like the slow rush of an ocean wave.

"Welcome, traveler! What brings you out so far?"

Jaina grinned in pure pleasure. "Why, just seeing what the dreams above the clouds are like!"

Jupiter laughed a sound that rang across the entire solar system.

"Would you like to see what I see? Come into my eye and I will show you the things that even I dream about."

Excited beyond measure, Jaina flew toward the planet. "Yes, please! I want to see!"

As she dove into the great eye it became like a perfect rainstorm surrounding her, only the rain was made of soft light.

Winds swirled about her in a choir older than humanity itself, welcoming her, buoying her on their sweet serenade.

Then the swirling clouds broke and she saw with the planet's great eye. In an instant, her gaze was cast across the cosmos, beyond the planets of the solar system with their great icy rings and pale colors.

She saw to distant stars, which burned with a halo of colors, serpentine "sun dogs" coiling gracefully around them, and the myriad kaleidoscope shapes that appeared in their fiery surfaces.

Each one was a lens for the dreams of distant places, shining a light into the beautiful expanse of space.

Her gaze swung again and she saw to a vast maroon cloud unfolding. It looked like a giant bird unfurling its wings, speckled with stars like diamonds studding its feathers.

Its great fiery plume slowly expanded, the whole nebula growing like an eagle spreading its wings for the flight across the vastness of the cosmos.

Points of brilliant light appeared around it in great reddish-white flashes, and in each, one was born a new world of dreams.

The birdlike nebula opened its beak and uttered a cry of creation, and from its throat flowed the stuff of which worlds were made. Dust, gases, and matter flowed forth in a flood so titanic it would blanket a world, spiraling together, a burning ember at its heart. More joined the cosmic deluge and more still, and in the heart of it all, a star was born from the very dreams of the universe.

The bird-nebula spread its wings further and flew from one end of space to the other, trailing pure magic from its wings.

Comets and belts of stars and spinning rings floated outward from its wake, each going on to seek yet more places to manifest celestial phenomena.

Jaina in Jupiter's eye blinked and then it looked further still, watching a star in its final brilliant moments before it burst.

Impossibly bright, it is light-filled the firmament. Each ray carried the wishes of all who had looked upon a star and wished, each one forming from Dreamtime to scatter across the universe.

New paths were born for those who dreamed to reach the most far-flung of destinations, forged by the light of the dying star.

Even its magnificent ending created new life, for itself and for others, by filling the universe with newfound hope and inspiration.

Beyond the supernova lay a band of similar stars suspended in white mist. The whole of the Milky Way galaxy stretched out before her.

Its beating heart was a bright white center around which the entire Dreamtime world spiraled, all sharing the same space and time.

For here, there were no barriers between time and thought, spirit and space, dream and cosmic law.

Nebulae unfolded in silent compositions that told of the birth of entire worlds. Stars emerged from the ether and grew into cosmic forges so hot that to strike upon them was to shape solar systems.

The majesty she witnessed expanding across the boundless universe was enough to forever touch Jaina's imagination.

Nothing she had ever dreamed prepared her for the scope and the power of the universe on this scale.

She swam in a vision of pure bliss borne upon the very spirit of the cosmos and felt its irresistible pull.

Cool blue stars glimmered in the clouds of reddish-white dust.

Planets swam through the great ocean of space, caught in the tides cast by the stars.

Comets soared through this like great travelers exploring worlds unknown.

The universal music reached from the very highest to the very smallest, leaving nothing untouched by its harmonies.

Light flowed across the known and unknown, hemmed by the dark of open space, a grand vision of timeless existence.

The most potent of possibilities collided with the least of impossibilities to bring forth the stuff of dreams and visions.

For each raindrop that fell upon an ocean, a star shone in the heavens and brought to light yet another facet of this incalculable grandness.

Jaina slept, completely enthralled by the visions of all that was and all that would one day exist, and how it sang from the very instruments of creation.
She felt her small part in that primordial music and she knew peace, oneness with the universe.

For only in a dream could someone know what it truly meant to be a part of it all, a wanderer in a place so incredible that it defied pure understanding, and yet never alone on the journey?
Every star in the universe shone its light upon her, and in turn, her every dream fed them. Every time she saw a star twinkle in the sky from that day forth, Jaina knew.
The stars were dreaming, too.

Travels

Through parallel dimensions
Travels in time and space
Seeking companionship without pretensions
Searching for a giver of much-needed advice
A keeper of secrets and dreams
Nothing else will suffice
Shall I find them running thru the park
Or perhaps getting lost on an adventure,
And ending up in an enchanted cave after dark
Through travels, I found a confidant and friend
A gentle, kindred soul
Who will travel unfettered through time, and space until the end

Time?

Does it seem that you are stuck in the past?
You know the times are good, but they won't last.
Do you feel that you've lived in this time before?
And no matter what you, do the die has already been cast...
Does it feel that strangers are all the friends you used to know
And you left them in the future to come and watch this show
Of all the things you did and the person you used to be
Do you feel this too, or is it just me
Perhaps its already happened before we ever began
Maybe time is just a spiral and we're all just dancers
Going around and round
jumping back and forth looking for some answers

Floating through Space

I am weightless, a celestial flyer

I float passed planets, rising higher
I somersault and spin
This vast universe where does it begin?
Galaxies in the distance, I observe
A meteor on a collision course, I must swerve
Tumbling where there is not up or down
Stars, shooting all around
I soar and I swoop, taking in the worlds unknown
From one of them imitates and otherworldly tone
That planet there with the multi-colored rings
It has a voice, with an eerie melody, it sings
Floating through space, I am but a traveling soul
All of this wonder and beauty must extol
When at last, to my bed I must finally return
I close my eyes and sigh, and for the stars, I yearn

Shooting Star

I once took a ride upon a shooting star
I traveled so fast and so far,
I heard each and every with as it was made
And watched every dream as it was displayed
I once took a ride across the midnight sky
Soaring with glee, as I pretend to fly
Basking in the star's fiery glow
I watched with wonder at each village below
I once took a ride through my window and into my bed
I felt the droop of my eye and the nod of my head
Then away again, I rode to the land of dreams
To remember that magic is sometimes more than it seems

Chapter 10: The Stunning World

Jane plunged into the water, feeling the unwieldy weight of her diving equipment leave her instantly. The water lifted the burden from her back and, as she adjusted to the breathing apparatus, her attention was placed squarely on herself.

Finally adjusting to the pressure, the shifting presence of the tank on her back, the pressure of her diving suit, and the pressure of the goggles on her face, she was able to look around at the stunning world around her.

She could see the other divers from her group plunging into the water around her, taking pictures with their waterproof cameras, taking in the wildlife that skittered and flowed beneath and around them, and marveling at this whole world that lay beneath the island where they had been vacationing.

Jane floated for a moment, looking into the deepening expanse that lay before her. As she stared into the distance, she could see the shimmering blue of the ocean darkening toward the horizon.

She didn't expect to be able to see so far ahead of her or that the water would look so calm from underneath the surface. She could see fish lazily ambling through the water, barely taking heed of, yet relying on the currents in it.

She made her way closer to the white sands that lay at the bottom of the ocean. The water wasn't terribly deep here, so she knew she could swim down to it without getting lost or putting herself out of her depth.

In the white sand, she saw many small shells and sensed a movement that came from the current that danced above. As she watched the sands arrhythmically moving, she saw a small crab pop up from beneath the surface and scuttle under a nearby rock.

She gawked at the life that teemed around her, swimming from place to place and admiring its beauty. As she did so, she found herself drifting further and further away from the boat that had brought them to the diving site. They were told they could go pretty far away from the site, but to stay close enough that you could still see at least one other diver.

She made sure she could see one diver as she continued looking for more pretty sights to see under the waves. As she hovered in the water, she swore she saw something whip across the floor beneath her. Slightly alarmed, but trying to keep her breathing even, she looked around to see if she could find the thing that had slipped past her.

Over the occasional hiss of her breathing apparatus, she heard the gentle swish of quick motion through the water behind her. She whipped her head around, but still heard nothing. Out of a sense of fear and self-preservation, Jane made her way back over to the group. She stayed with them until the session was over and uneventfully made her way back up onto the boat.

In her hotel room, she couldn't help but think about the presence that whipped around her in the water. She really had seen it there, right? It hadn't been some figment brought about by the heat from being on the beach all morning before her dive, had it? Either way, she needed to get back to the water to figure out what it was.

She looked out at the ocean from the balcony of her hotel room. She could see the spot where they had been diving that day. It was dark out, so there wasn't much of anything to see in that spot. The waves on the water were choppier than they had been in the afternoon and the wind had kicked up slightly.

She felt compelled to watch that spot in the ocean as the wind blew and the waves rolled. She was unable to take her eyes off the spot where they had been that afternoon, and he had also been unable to figure out how she knew that was where they had been. She hadn't even needed to think about it; she just knew that was the spot. As she pondered this, eyes transfixed on that spot, she saw something glowing beneath the surface. Something... big

She wanted to call the front desk and ask about the thing glowing in the ocean, but she couldn't bring herself to move from that spot. From the muscles in her forehead, all the way down to her pinky toes, she could not compel any muscle in her body to move even the slightest bit, as it would mean possibly interrupting her view of the brilliant light that blazed beneath the waves. She could swear, as she watched it, that it was getting brighter and larger at a pace that her eyes could barely process. It was slow but certain.

Her ears twitched as she watched the light. Was it... Singing? It sounded like a hum, a screech, a hymn, and a bell, all rolled into one song. It was not a cacophonous sound, though her mind seemed to insist that it ought to have been for all the elements that it contained. She was thankful that she couldn't will herself to move. Everything in her mind was screaming at her to jump over the railing of her balcony and into the ocean to see what was calling to her from the deep.

Before she could make heads or tails of all the things that were going on at that moment, everything went dark. The song, the ocean, the light, the room, the city below... Everything, All at once, the waves in the ocean completely subsided and settled into a calm, glassy surface that reflected the moon, which somehow also seemed muted. She felt the tension in her muscles release suddenly and before she could compensate, she tumbled to the floor, losing consciousness on the way down.

She awoke the next morning to the sun shining through the open balcony door, birds calling, and calm waves crashing periodically on the beach below. She was still on the floor, wearing her clothes from the evening before. She picked herself up off the floor and made herself take a shower, get some coffee, and get dressed. Once she had taken care of herself, she would get some answers about what had been going on the night before.

She entered the lobby and saw that it was business as usual for the guests and employees in the resort. People were milling about, asking questions about gratuities, breakfast, check-in times, and scheduled tours. She peered around to see if she found anyone that looked anywhere near as unsettled as she felt but there didn't seem to be anyone who fit that description.

She walked up to the concierge desk to talk to the sharply dressed woman there that wore a bright, happy smile.

"Excuse me," she started.

"Yes, madam; how can I be of service?"

"Do you know anything about the blackout that happened last night? What was it that caused it?"

"I'm sorry? Did you lose power in your room last night? I can ask the front desk if there were any interruptions they might know about."

"No, I mean the blackout in the whole... Did the city not lose power last night?"

"No, ma'am, I don't think there was anything like that here last night. Would you like me to ask the front desk?" Jane's mind was racing.

"Oh... No, that's okay. Thank you." Jane didn't wait for a response before she went back into the elevator and ran back up to her room. She changed into her swimsuit and ran back downstairs and out to the beach.

She asked about scuba tours that would be going back out to that spot, but the instructor said that there wouldn't be any tours that day due to a family emergency for the instructor. The man at the booth was simply there for equipment rental.

She rented the equipment she needed and suited up, heading right for the spot where she had been diving the day before. The spot where she had seen that impossibly large light, how had no one seen it? How had no one reported on anything that had happened the night before? Had she suffered some sort of heat exhaustion that made her imagine the entire thing? Maybe this solo vacation had been a mistake after all.

Once she was certain she had all her gear on properly, she dove into the water off the platform that jutted out into the water. She looked around for any sign of the presence that she had felt the day before. At first, there wasn't anything strange going on in the water around her. In the silent calm of the water, she began to feel silly. Maybe she had just chased a complete illusion all the way out here and maybe there never was anything strange in the water at all.

She turned around to make her way back toward the ladder that extended into the water from the platform off of which she had jumped. As she swam toward the ladder, she heard it. Her blood ran cold and she felt the hot tingle of alarm pulse through her body. She stopped swimming and listened for a moment. When she heard nothing further, she turned very slowly to look at what had made the noise.

Nothing, before she could feel anything at all about the lack of a presence in the water with her, she saw it. Something barreling through the water from leagues away, it was impossibly swift; ignoring any resistance the water should have posed. As it dashed toward her, it kept its eyes fixed on her.

Her muscles once again refused to move in any measure as she met its eyes. Dear Lord, she thought. It's massive.

Its eyes seemed miles wide as its gaze held hers. In seconds, the monstrosity covered an incredible distance. Jane tried to brace herself for impact as it closed in, but she could only float, powerless. Its immense mouth opened as it got mere feet from her. Its teeth were jagged and craggy. Each one would have been deadly on its own if it had been wielded by a person. Lined into the gaping maw before her, they were the gateway to oblivion.

As the darkness enveloped her, she could swear that she heard humming… Humming that also seemed like a screech, a hymn, with just a hint of bells. My God, it's beautiful, she thought.

Chapter 11: Alone on the Moon

Before we begin this journey downwards into the deepest realms of our subconscious, let us take a minute to physically and mentally and spiritually acclimate ourselves into being with an awareness of our inner sanctum, our internal workings. We will begin by going to a place of comfort, ideally a bed, or a very comfortable reclining chair, and we will relax our bodies to the furthest extent possible. Now, close your eyes, staying firmly on your back, with your arms relaxed at your sides and your legs rested downwards. Take one deep breath in your nostrils, counting slowly to four, and one deep breath out, through your nostrils again, counting slowly to four. Breathe in the breath of the spirit and breathe out the stress of the day. Now is the time to rest. Become aware of nothing but the air flowing through your nostrils, envision a steady flowing stream, smooth inhalations, and exhalations; your body becomes weightier and more relaxed with each passing cycle of breath. Allow your thoughts to become completely still. You focus on your core, your solar plexus, allowing your thoughts to flow outwards past your vision until they escape your being while only holding and retaining the pure awareness of spirit holy serenity of the mind and body. Breathe in, one, two, three, four, then breathe out, one, two, three, four, each breath becoming slower. One... two... three... four... One... two... three... four... One... two... three... four... One... two... three... four... One... two... three... four... One... two... three... four... Continue this pattern of breath, expanding, and sink deeper into yourself, becoming a voyeur of your own still, relaxed body, lost in time. Become lost in this experience as you journey further into the trance, and prepare for the road we are about to embark upon. Draw further and further away from your still, lying body, and into the realm of imagination, where images grow, the land of dreams that you are about to become one with. Erase your mind of all that is within it currently, and prepare the landscape for a new and fresh experience, in the farther reaches of reality. One... two... three... four... inhale... One... two... three... four... exhale... One... two... three... four... inhale... One... two... three... four... exhale... Now, with your mind, body, and spirit rested, entranced, and fertile, let us begin.

You find yourself on the surface of the moon. You are alone. You move your body. Everything feels ethereally heavy as if you are as big as the universe, yet light, as if there is barely any pull towards the ground. You jump up and stay up, and fall slowly to the ground. You scream. No sound is heard. You scream again, as loud as you can. All the rage you have ever felt, any fear or any negative feeling that has ever crossed your path in this eternal life comes pouring out of you in one giant scream. Yet there is nothing. There is no mark made on this atmosphere by your pain, for there is no atmosphere, for you are alone, on the moon. With the silent scream, go your memories. Just as your scream went silent on this surface, meaningless and less than it ever did in your known reality back on planet earth, too does any negative feeling that came with it. Everything begins to evaporate here, as now there is only you, alone, weightless and free. You jump up and down and up and down, making incredible bounds with each leap. You are floating, flying, across a surface hitherto unimaginable by the average human. Very few people have ever been here, and you are now one of them. Whereas they had to wear very large and heavy and intricate suits, guard against the elements, and breathe, you are naked. You can breathe effortlessly as if the deprivation of oxygen has been replaced with a breath of spirit that charges your entire body in an even greater sense than the oxygen of the earth. Every breath you take is like ten breaths that activate parts of your body that you have never felt before. You are leaping, incredibly, up and up into the air, then, leisurely, falling ever so slowly down. You kick, and wave, and flip around. It is like being in the middle of the ocean, yet vacant, and clear, and black. Grey rock spreads before you as far as you can see, in every direction. Gigantic mountains give way into even larger craters as if the pores and hairs on the skin of some great stone deity. You feel the vibration from this deity course through you, silent, with no sound. Yet there is a feeling, and this feeling, in its own right, is louder than any sound you have ever heard, or could ever hope to make. It is pure spirit, charging through you. All around you is black, and stars, closer than they have ever been in your memory. The stars are larger, like fireflies, floating in the pure black sky. And there is the earth, your memories, now so very far away, as to be almost meaningless. But it is beautiful. You feel so removed from it now, yet you can bask in its beauty in a way you never thought possible. The great blue planet, a blue orb unto itself, alone in the cosmos, so far away from any neighbor; so far away from you. You think about your life there. Like picking up a handful of sand, the grains slowly pass through your fingers. There is much subjectivity in life and such a changing of being. Your environment so defines your environment, yet your environment is so temporary and so prone to change. What you know as life on earth couldn't exist here naturally. That being the biology, the skin, the flesh, the blood, the organs, everything that comprises what you have hitherto known to be life. Yet, here you are, beyond all this physiological being, a being of pure spirit, boundless, defying all laws of physics, transcending the existence that you had previously been indebted to, becoming something new, unknown, yet knowing itself, through the experience, feeling mysterious yet familiar. With infinite of leaps behind you, the earth has come and gone a million times, and you come upon the base of one of those great, gray mountains that had been in the distance. Time has passed into oblivion, yet you are still here. No hunger, no pain, no fear. You are to traverse up this mountain; you know it in your heart. You take the first leap, then the second, and you're climbing, climbing at the speed of light. Dust and rocks fly behind you, with every landing, with every spring of the foot. You feel as if the whole mountain could crumble beneath you, so you become gentle more and more, careful, as it is your responsibility, if you so choose, to keep this mountain as it exists, tall, reaching up from the surface into the heavens it came from. Softly, you continue up the mountain, making large strides, until, there you are, at the top. You feel as if you might just float off into space, but some small force is keeping your feet tethered to the ground if they want to be. You twirl around, your arms out in front of you, and you can see what seems to be the moon's entire surface, even though that would be impossible. You see the edges rounding down into the globe, each crater, every lump of rock, every other mountain, yet this is the largest, and you are the master of it. You jump up as high as you can, and it seems as if you are a mile above the peak. You twirl, and twirl, as slow as you can, spinning in slow motion as you float like a feather, slowly, slowly, back down to the peak. The tip of your foot touches the highest point, and you balance there, forever, the earth coming and going and coming and going as you stand in this balance, effortlessly, free, nothing pushing or pulling on your being, just you, still, there. After several lifetimes, you feel the urge to go back down the mountainside, so you roll forward, and begin to tumble, like a tumbling weed in the wind, all the way down. With every bounce, you are ten feet in the air, and, before you know it, you have reached the familiar plateau of the surface, and there you are, with one final bounce, rested on the flat of the moon. You lay there for as long as you were at the top, several more lifetimes, still, in the lone, empty, black, and white void. There is nothing. And then you fall asleep.

Chapter 12: The Wisdom Search

"As I read this and begin to drift comfortably asleep, I don't know whether I will find myself drifting asleep more to the sound of my voice or the words I read, or perhaps to the spaces between the words. And as I drift comfortably asleep I'll just read this story to myself."

So, as you listen to me and you comfortably begin to fall asleep, I don't know whether you will find yourself drifting comfortably to sleep to the sounds of my words, to the spaces between my words, or just listening along to my voice in the background as you fall asleep. And while you fall asleep I am just going to tell you a story about a man who enjoyed going out to sea.

Every year he would go on a trip on a boat. His favourite thing was to swim with humpback whales. Every year he would go out on a boat, he would go out to sea on that boat and he would sit on that boat in diving gear and wait. And he would wait patiently and quietly, listening to the water lapping on the side of the boat, feeling the gentle rocking of the boat as he just gazes out over the water, feeling the sea breeze on his skin, noticing what the sky looks like, gazing out towards the horizon, scanning around the horizon, scanning the water for signs of the humpback whales arriving. And every year those humpback whales seem to arrive in this location.

And so, he just sits calmly and patiently and waits and not only does he like diving with the humpback whales, but he finds the entire experience calming and relaxing, just having patience, nothing to think about or worry about. Just waiting and relaxing. And then after some time, as the sun passes across the sky, he sees a little cloud appear from the ocean. And then the dark back of a humpback whale slides just above the surface of the water and back under again, so he drives the boat closer to the whales. And the closer he gets, the more he sees of what is there. He notices that there is an adult humpback whale and a juvenile humpback whale and he sees how calmly they are just swimming through the water. He drops the anchor and he drops into the water. He can feel that water flow into his wetsuit as he dives down under the water in his scuba gear. And he can see the size of those whales, see their slow graceful movements, hearing the whale calls. Just watching as those whales gracefully swim passed and watching how those whale's eyes appear to be so inquisitive, with such curiosity. And how the juvenile whale seems to want to come over to him and explore him. And the adult whale just keeps that juvenile at a bit of distance while assessing the diver and only after some assessing does the adult allow the juvenile and themselves to move closer.

They swim close enough for the diver to reach out with their hand and while their hand is outstretched, the juvenile swims in and rubs itself against his hand. And like all his past experiences, he feels this experience is an incredible experience, a moving experience, showing such intelligence in these whales, such love from the whales. He turns himself around weightlessly in the water, to keep tracking those whales as they swim comfortably around him. He enjoys this time in the water. Being in the water weightless with these whales, time seems to stand still. And after a while the whales take a deep breath and dive and he watches as they swim deeper and deeper and disappear out of sight. He then goes back to the boat, gets on the boat and steers the boat back to shore loving the experience he has just had.

And back on the shore, he goes back to the caravan that he is staying in, he always drives down here in a VW camper van so he goes back to the camper van he is staying in. He sits down and keeps a journal of his experiences. Not just a journal of the acts that he did and the behaviours, but a journal of his feelings, of how the experience made him feel and what that means to him. And then, after writing his journal he sets up a camp just outside the caravan, just somewhere he can have something to eat on the seashore, a little campfire. And he enjoys the evening setting in, hearing the waves lashing on the shore, on the sand. Birds off in the distance, just sitting there enjoying the evening. Seeing the last of the suns' rays disappear and the stars in the sky. And as the evening draws on, he puts out the campfire, goes back into his camper van and settles down for the night to sleep. And as he drifts comfortably asleep, so he begins to dream and while he begins to dream, he begins to have a dream of himself sitting on a rose, sliding down a rose petal towards the centre of the rose and feeling the waxy touch of the petal under his hands as he slides and finding this feeling comfortable and safe and secure. The beautiful scent, the soft feeling of the waxy petal and he knows this dream has something to do with his daily experience. And he goes with the dream. And then he pops through the centre of the rose and finds himself sat at a desk in a chateau surrounded by woodland and mountains and finds that his hand is automatically writing as he gazes down at it and sees himself writing something unusual, he sees that he is writing some kind of a story.

He has this sense that he is writing a novel and he gets to a point where he gets drawn into that novel, into a scene where somebody is on a motorbike, going off-road, going around the outside of a mountain, following a mountain pass, following a dirt track. Riding that motorbike higher and higher up into the mountains. And he continues with the scene and there are a few areas where the motorbike skids and then catches the ground again and speeds off even faster and jumps at some areas and the bike is under full control of the motorcyclist. And that motorbike travels all the way to the top of the mountain. And the person on the motorbike is like a treasure hunter. And they are hunting for treasure that is somewhere here on the mountain and the person continues to write and as he continues to write he continues to be absorbed and drawn into this story, drawn into this story as this character discovers a temple high up here in this mountain.

And he picks a lock on the door to get into the temple, he walks into the temple and goes from the windy mountain's edge, to silence in the temple. He lights a torch and begins to explore in the temple and while he is exploring in the temple with the torch, so he can hear his footsteps echoing. He searches down one corridor and lights some torches as he goes and then searches down another corridor and then another. Noticing the way that his shadow and the light flickers on the walls, searching corridor after corridor. Until eventually, he comes to a dead end and at that dead end he sees what looks like a trap door on the ground. He prises open the trap door and climbs down a ladder going deeper and deeper under the temple and as he climbs deeper and deeper under the temple, so he realises he is climbing deeper and deeper down into the mountain, until eventually he comes out in a cave. And it appears to be a natural cave, it's not a man made cave. He thinks that maybe the temple was built over the cave on purpose. And he continues to explore this cave. And while he is exploring the cave, he starts to hear dripping water and gradually he starts to hear the distant sound of a waterfall and he continues exploring the cave. And while he is exploring the cave he is looking for some sign of a huge lost diamond, a legendary diamond.

And everything led him to this place and so he continues exploring and while exploring he finds a tunnel from the cave that looks man made and so he follows that tunnel and goes deeper and deeper until it comes out in a room and at the far side of that room is a huge locked door and he picks that lock and enters the room and in the middle of the room is a pedestal with a huge diamond sitting on it, lit up by natural light that seems to be channeled to the centre of the room through ice from the outside. And he goes over to the diamond and his plan is to take the diamond and then sell it, but as he reaches the diamond he sees a book. He picks up the book and starts reading and as he starts reading so he learns that this diamond is placed here to bring peace to the land and that there is darkness that will be unleashed if this diamond gets removed. And anyone who discovers this diamond has to look inside themselves and decide what is more important, peace across the land, keeping the darkness at bay, or having the diamond and making lots of money? And he thinks about it. He doesn't know what this darkness is, he can't imagine a real darkness, that would be the thing of legends and myths, so it must be a legend or a myth, it can't be real. The book ends by saying that he is to put his hands on either side of the pedestal where there are two symbols and to close his eyes and that will teach him that everything in this book is true. He thinks to himself that it all sounds ridiculous, but it takes no effort to put your hands on the side of something and to close your eyes for a moment, to prove that it is ridiculous.

So, he puts his hands on either side of the pedestal and he closes his eyes and initially he doesn't feel anything and then he starts feeling a tingling at his hands, that starts in his fingers, or perhaps his palm and eventually starts moving up to his wrists, his arms, his shoulders and in to his body and a warmth, a comfort and he has a sense of a light, a purple light, as if it is given off by the diamond in front of him. He can see it with his eyes closed, he can sense that purple light shining on his face, passing into his head, his body, absorbing into him, this purple light, passing in to him, filling him up with this purple light. And he starts to have a feeling of serenity, of peace, of love, of wonder and curiosity, a sense of a connection with the world around him, a sense of what is important. And he finds it a powerful, emotive experience. And then he removes his hands from the pedestal and in a moment the experience passes and he opens his eyes and he is just there with that pedestal with that diamond and he realises that the diamond needs to stay where it is and needs to be protected. And he leaves and seals the entrance to that room and he leaves and seals every entrance behind him and leaves that mountaintop temple and seals the door and then motorbike's back down the mountain with that serene feeling, that learning, that knowledge he gained that will stay with him forever.

And the writer had this feeling that the story was coming closer to an end, as the man found himself with the petals falling down around him, gently floating down to the ground, as he was sat in the middle of these giant rose petals, just falling around him, comfortably, calmly, as he drifted from this dream into a deeper more comfortable, healing, relaxing, sleep.

Chapter 13: At the Beach

Before we begin this journey downwards into the deepest realms of our subconscious, let us take a minute to physically and mentally and spiritually acclimate ourselves into being with awareness of our inner-sanctum, our internal workings.

We will begin by going to a place of comfort, ideally a bed, or a very comfortable reclining chair, and we will relax our bodies to the furthest extent possible. Now, close your eyes, staying firmly on your back, with your arms relaxed at your sides and your legs rested downwards.

Take one deep breath in, through your nostrils, counting slowly to four, and one deep breath out, through your nostrils again, counting slowly to four. Breathe in the breath of the spirit and breathe out the stress of the day.

Now is the time to rest. Become aware of nothing but the air flowing through your nostrils; envision a steady flowing stream, smooth inhalations and exhalations, your body become weightier and more relaxed with each passing cycle of breath.

Allow your thoughts to become completely still, as you focus on your core, your solar plexus, allowing your thoughts to flow outwards past your vision until they escape your being, while only holding and retaining the pure awareness of spirit, the holy serenity of the mind and body.

Breathe in, one, two, three, four, then breathe out, one, two, three, four, each breath becoming slower.

One... two... three... four...

One... two... three... four...

One... two... three... four...

One... two... three... four...

One... two... three... four...

Continue this pattern of breath, expanding, and sink down deeper into yourself, becoming a voyeur of your own still, relaxed body, lost in time.

Become lost in this experience as you journey further into the trance, and prepare for the road we are about to embark upon. Draw further and further away from your still, lying body, and into the realm of imagination, where images grow, the land of dreams that you are about to become one with.

Erase your mind of all that is within it currently, and prepare the landscape for a new and fresh experience, in the farther reaches of reality.

One... two... three... four... inhale...

One... two... three... four... exhale...

One... two... three... four... inhale...

One... two... three... four... exhale...

Now, with your mind, body, and spirit rested totally, entranced, and fertile, let us begin.

You have taken a day off to spend at the beach.

You are alone, and feel totally comfortable in your own skin. Around you are large crowds, but they feel very far away from you, and their presence does not overwhelm you in the slightest.

There is a bubble around you, and, in fact, the presence of the crowd is uplifting, both in its juxtaposition with yourself, and in its own self-sustainability. These crowds of people are happy and loving and having the greatest times of their lives, and they are totally independent of you, and need nothing from you, as you need nothing from them.

There is a great peace in this that you feel, a calm that there could be so much right in the world that exists totally without any need from you. It is inspiring and uplifting, and makes you feel free.

The presence of the crowds does absolutely nothing to affect your ability to enjoy the natural pleasures of the beach. It seems as if the crowd has parted perfectly to allow you the best view possible of the shore and the horizon. You wonder how far out the water is visible. It could be one mile, or a hundred. To you, what you are seeing seems infinite, and infinitely calm. You feel as if you could walk across the beach and into the water and drift forever into the void of this great blue mass, and there would be no end in sight.

At the edge of what is visible to you, the sky opens up, being an even greater and holier chasm, the abyss of the sea spread exponentially into the universe. It is amazing to you to watch these two divine forces, reflections of each other, connect and touch and embrace.

It is you, yourself, embracing the infinite. The sand around you, likewise, is infinite, being an infinite number of grains. Every handful that you pick up and allow to pass through your fingers is infinity, a universe of universes.

You are humbled by the sheer number of particles that make up this small space within your bubble, and in its close proximity your mind wanders exponentially to the infinities lying elsewhere, within the other infinities, the small, personal spaces that make up our existence, and the endless number of spaces there can be.

You are melting into the ground through your beach towel, as every particle of you intermingles with the endless particles in the sand, and every particle in your soul floats into the breeze towards the shore, interspersing through the waters until they end their journey at the horizon, at which point the dust will float up through the heavens, and eternity.

You are melting, sinking, and your mind is leaving your body. Time slows down inside of your bubble as it speeds up among those crowds that had once been around you, now light-years away. Generations come and go among the beach crowds, as you remain perfectly still, and content, a part of something greater than yourself, yet which is only great because of yourself, the infinity.

An eternity passes and you are back on the beach. You get up, the beach air bringing new life back into your lungs, and your blood, and your body, and your mind. Your eyes gaze anew upon the sight as you make your way towards the water, through the path that has been cleared by the universe through this large, intangible crowd that seems totally unaware of your presence. It is an infinite and joyous walk to the shore, and feels like walking towards the light, towards the afterlife.

You feel the sand become wet at your feet, and where the particles once brushed up into the crevices of your feet and fell through, now they are molding into you, a larger mass, bonded by the water, each step leaving an impression in the sand which welcomes you with open arms, like a slipper that fits just right.

Eventually, your feet feel the total submersion into the water, and the sand totally beneath. Instantly, you are connected most tangibly to the entire whole.

Whereas you were always a part of this abyss, now it has awakened within you tenfold, and upon first touch you feel the water connecting to the sky at the horizon, connecting to the heavens above. There is only blue, a great, blue abyss, a serenity that perpetuates outwards for eternity. You continue, and continue to be submerged.

As the water goes up above your waistline, you feel your entire body become weightless. You look back and see the crowds, and it feels as if you are in space looking back down onto the planet from which you came. In a beautiful way, the people on the beach seem like insects, and you feel totally removed from any part of them.

The void behind you is what you feel the closest kinship with; it's infinite stretches and unending silence and space. You fall back into the water, and as it touches your head your mind melts away into this endless sea of blue.

You are now flowing, totally weightless, into the abyss. You float for what seems like hours, then days, then weeks, then months, then years, then a lifetime, then further generations down, but it is only a second. This continues for a long while before you have reached that horizon, that point that you saw back on the beach where the blue of the waters transcended into the blue of the sky.

With this meeting, you transcend as well, as your entire being transmutes into the air, becoming the glowing golden clouds of the sunset. You are as large as the entire visible sky, looking down at the place you came from, glowing golden between the earth and the heavens.

For an eternity, the sun sits at the horizon, projecting you onto the clouds, the golden glow of your soul.

As it fades, your consciousness fades, and the whole of your golden glow becomes broken into infinite pieces, becoming the multitude of stars in the sky.

Now you are in space, divided amongst the cosmos, neither here nor there, in infinite black. You are totally still, you are the night sky, and you are asleep.

Chapter 14: In the Bar

Every time Mark placed his hand against the bottle of beer, and he felt the coldness of it, something tingled in his being. From the back of his head, through his spine, and ending in the middle of his butt. That had been the only refreshing experience that he had known for the past three months since Lizzy left him. Shocked? Yeah, he was shocked that Lizzy could leave. Yet had he expected it. The warning signs had come, they were flashing in his eyes. At least he could not deny that one. She was unaffectionate, she could not be satisfied, and she increased the tempo of her nagging, hell, he could even say by a hundred percent. It was all just unexplainable, and he wished things would get better. Just like most stories like this, they never did. So, he just waited for what would unavoidably come, Lizzy, leaving him alone in the darkness that had consumed his soul with the prolonged times of strive and the likes. This is why there could be no other thing that he could rely on than on this fragile bottle, which he knew would one day send him crashing to the floor. Why he kept on to that too, no one could tell.

"When are you going to quit?" Clark asked him.

"I don't know, man. I just don't know," Mark replied.

That was the most real person he had still, but he walked away. Clark could not tell of any way he could have helped Mark. Any light that was truly going to set him at liberty would have to come from deep within himself.

"Help me, Lord," Mark muttered more often than ever.

On this evening, he had said the same words, while he yet turned to the green bottles at a bar. But on this evening, he could not deny, there had been a great restlessness over his being, all over. There was nothing he felt that he could do about it, but he knew the way to his favorite bar, and that was just where he went. If the universe ever did its work, or say, something like destiny, that must have been what was at work that evening. He met Tom, a lazy folk that walked into the bar. He had taken a couple of beers and seemed terrified. Frantic, he began searching all over for where his purse had been. He looked so much in panic, that Mark's attention, even in his depression had just been drawn to him. Mark was halfway through his drunkenness. At this stage, he could still comprehend to an extent of decent reasoning, but the speaking part was not so much what he could put up with.

"You little runt, you had better bring out my money or I am squeezing you till there is no life in you," the angry barman had said.

Why was he being so unfair? Could he not see that the little man had truly lost his wallet, and who knows what with it?

"I swear to you, man, I swear to you, I do not know where my wallet is. It was just here right now, right here with me. I swear it. I think I have been robbed!" Tom yelled, enough for every person who had been in that bar to hear him loud and clear.

"Every thief swears he is not a thief. I stole my wife's money last night. I swore on my mama's grave I had not even been at home at the time she speculated," a drunken man yelled from another side of the bar.

His comment was accompanied by the laughter of others. The barman did not seem to enjoy the rowdiness of the bar, but he had his eyes stuck to the little thief. Mark took his time to examine him for the first time. He seemed a teenage or a little above it. Say he was twenty-one or twenty-two.

"I can swear I have heard of this kind of trick before. You drink and you don't pay and you fake the loss of your wallet. Fucking loser. You are going to pay every dime or you will lose bones in your body tonight. I swear that to you," the barman said, sounding angrier. He had been a really big man, even he seemed larger than the regular size. At this point, he seemed to be advancing towards Mark, and there was no smile on his face.

"Leave him alone, I will pay," Mark said in his drunken tone.

"What?" the barman and Tom echoed together in unbelief.

"I will pay for the lad. Let him be. Add his bills to mine," Mark repeated, as he pushed a wad of cash towards the barman.

"Thank you, sir," Tom said, shyly, towards Mark.

"You're welcome," Mark mouthed at Tom.

"You lucky beast, now get out of my bar," the barman said, angrily.

As Tom tried to get himself together, preparing to scamper out of the bar, Mark spoke again.

"Nah! Let the lad stay with me. Let him drink as much as he wants to. The bill is on me," Mark said.

Tom looked at the barman and gave a sheepish smile. Furious, the barman slammed a rolled towel against the slab and walked away. Tom, at this point, made fresh orders from the other barman and he sipped slowly and gracefully. There had been silence between them, in what seemed to be like through the entire bar. Tom passed cursory looks towards Mark and wished he could do something, or better still, say something to make him know that he was grateful for what he had done. Mark saved him the stress by speaking first.

"You did not have a wallet, did you?" Mark asked.

"Sir?" Tom pretended not to have heard the question.

"I did silly things like that as a kid too, you know." Mark continued.

"I am sorry sir, but sometimes, it just gets also crazy that a guy needs more beer than he can afford, you know?" Tom replied.

"Were those not the things that made us light enough to think we literally floated through life, being weighed down by nothing?" Mark asked.

Tom turned to examine Mark for a moment as though he could not believe the things that he was saying.

"Exactly sir, exactly," Tom finally replied.

They continued drinking and did so for a short while.

"You seem like the married kind, are you?" Tom asked.

"Is that a pleasant way of saying that I look stressed?" Mark asked, laughing.

"Perhaps," Tom replied.

"Well, I am not married," Mark said.

"Then what brings you here, why do you want to float?" Tom asked.

"Escape," Mark replied.

"What from, if I may ask?" Tom askes.

Tom went wordless for a short while. Meticulously, he took sips at his glass.

"Boy, I was once like you, you know, free and flying. Then I met this woman that I know I truly loved. Then things began to fly high for me," Mark began to explain.

He put his hand in the air, like a bird and he glided from the point of the table to higher and higher.

"Then all of a sudden, dash! I crash down like a little bird," Mark concluded.

"What struck you in the air, truly?" Tom asked.

"What do you mean? I just told you a woman I loved left me and that affected me so bad. What do you mean what struck me, kid?" Mark asked.

"Most times, we know what happens to us, but what we do not investigate is how we let what happened to us, really happen to us," Tom said.

Mark dropped his glass and looked into his eyes in unbelief.

"I swear, I have never heard a drunken man so wise," Mark said, laughing.

Tom burst out in laughter too and soon, they were both laughing out loud.

"Tell me though, what struck you. How did you give in?" Tom asked again.

"You know, it was obvious we were headed to that direction of things, but I kept hoping, holding on, something like that. You know. I kept wishing, even though I knew all was gone. Maybe that was not the crime," Mark replied.

"What was the real crime then?" Tom asked.

"Waiting to be loved, not knowing I had the power to love myself," Mark replied as he raised the glass again to his lips.

Tom gave no response to what he had said. He seemed melancholic, his face reddened after a while.

"What is wrong with you, man?" Mark asked.

"I remember when my mama died. Every single evening, for two months, I walked up to her grave to weep. I looked at the gravestone, looked at her picture in it and just cried. It was a festival of sorrow, every single day for sixty days or more," Tom explained.

"Oh, I am sorry about that," Mark replied.

"Then one day, I come to realize that I was drilling through the same sore that I hoped would heal. I discovered that deep down I did not want it to heal, I wanted to feel the pain over and over again. I thought that was the best way to keep alive her memory in me. I thought it was love, but I got to the realization that love was more. Love meant keeping ourselves strong too, and not feeling the worst for those we loved. Love meant letting go too. Then I chose to let go. It took a while, but I let go in the end," Tom explained.

Mark was silent.

"This is no philosophical shit, man. I mean it from the depth of my being, man. Let go. Walk by, walk past. That is life. We walk by things and people, if they are not meant to be with us, we must learn to walk past," Tom said.

"I hear you, kid," Mark replied, sober.

"Holding on to the blade that cut us would stitch no wound, man," Tom said.

In Mark's mind, he knew that it was true, everything that Tom said to him.

"I want you to go home, get yourself together, and be the best of you that you can be. All of this is for yourself. You have tried so long in being the best for others; you must put in the same energy for yourself now," Tom continued.

Mark thought about everything that Tom had said to him in that instance. He observed Tom as he hurriedly gulped down what was left of his beer mug, then he stood up to go.

"I have got to go, man," Tom said.

"But why, there is still much more to drink," Mark said, surprised.

"Perhaps. But I drink to enjoy and not to die. I have got no worries to drown," Tom said, patting Mark on the back as he walked away.

Mark wished after Tom had walked away, that he had gotten his phone number. Talking to someone of that kind was going to do the trick for him, at least, over a measured period. He had heard what he needed to hear, and what he needed to do was laid out there, crystal clear in his heart. It was time for him to walk past.

After that evening, Mark met Tom several times. It had been times of great talks as usual. However, after a while, he had stopped seeing him in the bar or anywhere around. Tom had moved, somehow. It was Mark's time to push through, but he discovered that Tom had given him the little strength that he needed to make a beautiful possibility out of that. Yes, Mark pulled through; he won, like every human was designed to win the conflicts of their souls. He knew that truly, things were made for us, and not us for them. The experiences of our lives are merely to teach us, not drag us on the streets of life as hopeless beings. Mark found the winner in himself after that evening, will you?

Chapter 15: The Lemonade

The anticipation overcomes me and I feel my hot, wet pussy throbbing in the middle of the night. I slip out of my tiny lacey underwear and toss them onto the floor. I slowly move my hand towards my pulsating pussy. I know that I won't take long to orgasm because I'm basically already there. Suddenly, I hear a loud noise coming from my front door. My sexual panting turns into pants of fear. I have no idea what that noise might be and I spring out of bed to find out. I quickly make it to my front window. I get the nerve to peer through my blinds to take a look. The entrance light is off but the moonlight shines brightly on a huge dog. It had run up next to my front door and had broken a ceramic flower pot that my best friend Laurie gave me. That explained the loud noise. I decided to check on the dog. I opened the front door slowly hoping there wouldn't be a weirdo there with the dog. Nobody was there. The dog was alone. I bent over to check the tag dangling from its collar when I suddenly felt a very quick shot of cool air. I jumped out of bed up so quickly when I heard the loud noise that I forgot to slip my panties on. The cool air hitting my bare, smooth, pink pussy felt awesome and got me even hotter. I inspected the dog tag thoroughly and started to memorize the phone number on it when suddenly I was startled by the noise of loud steps. I gasped quickly as I saw a shadow creep up behind me. "I'm so sorry I scared you and I apologize for my dog. I just moved into the neighborhood last week and my dog got out from the backyard. He's been gone all day. I was driving home late from work and he ran right in front of my car so I decided to stop and see where he ran to." I knew this guy had gotten a glimpse of my glistening pussy by the way he looked at me from head to toe and by how he couldn't quite look me in the eye as we spoke. "That's ok! I understand. The loud noise just scared the fuck out of me! I'm Alexa, by the way," I said as I tried to hold my short silk night gown down over my thighs as the cool wind blew. "Hi, I'm Bryce, your new neighbor from down the street." As we shook hands, I noticed some small drops of blood on the front porch. "Oh my God, I think your dog may be hurt. Why don't you come inside and check him out? It's a little chilly out here," I told Bryce. "Are you sure that's ok?" he asked. "Yes, of course," I said as I opened the door, lead them in, and went to look for a first aid kit. As Bryce made his way into my home, I noticed that he was very attractive and very, very muscular and well built. He was wearing a white long sleeve shirt and black slacks. It was obvious that he had not made it home from work yet so I knew his story was true. He rolled up his sleeves and started inspecting his dog as I sat on the loveseat next to him. I was very curious about how he would act knowing that I wasn't wearing any panties. Would he make a comment or just overlook it in a gentlemanly manner? At this point, I was so attracted to this almost-stranger named Bryce that I really wished he would make a comment about my "lack of panties". Then I would have a reason to show him more of me. "How long have you lived here?" he asked. He didn't let me answer and instead added more. "My ex-wife and I had to sell the house to settle our divorce and here I am." Ohhhhhh baby, YES!! He's freshly divorced and needs a good FUCK!! My pussy juices start flowing and I respond quickly. "I'm sorry about your divorce. I'm sure things will be better now." "Well, they are much better now that I have met you.

You are absolutely gorgeous!" "Awww...thanks." I tell him. "Would you like something to drink? I have tea and lemonade. " "I would love some, thank you," he said. I get up from the loveseat and walk to the kitchen. My nightgown is short enough that I know he got a very good look at my ass sticking out from underneath as I walked towards the refrigerator. I turn to catch him looking and giggle. "I'm so sorry. I don't mean to stare but I just can't keep my eyes off you. I think you have a great ass. I'm sure your boyfriend is very proud to have such a beautiful girl." I opened the fridge and bent over to get the carafe of lemonade. "oh, I don't have a boyfriend," I yelled out to make sure he heard me. As I stepped back from the fridge, I felt Bryce right behind me. "I was hoping to hear that because you have made me so fucking hard," he whispered as he grabbed my waist from behind. He started kissing my neck gently as he took the lemonade carafe from my hand and placed it on the granite counter. He stopped and asked, "Do you want me as much as I want you?" I appreciate him for asking. Here was a true gentleman that would love to get to know. I didn't answer his question but instead just pulled him near and started kissing him deeply. He was amazing. His tongue explored my mouth as I started to unbuckle his pants. His big hands moved up and down my back as he turned me back around. He pulled my golden hair aside and started to nibble on the back of my neck. That drove me absolutely crazy! He slipped his hands under my nightgown and cupped my huge DD breasts. He grabbed my hard nipples and started to pinch them gently as I quivered at his every touch. He wasn't wearing any clothes by now and I could feel his full-blown erection as I backed up into it. I moaned at his touch as his hands went on their own adventure. He slipped his hands down to my hot pussy and started to work his magic on my pulsating clit. I was very wet already and wanted him NOW! But Bryce wouldn't have it. He wanted to make love to me not just FUCK me. This told me that he was the loving type...a good guy. He's someone that I would have loved to have met sooner. Not now that I was about to move half-way across the country. Things didn't matter at this moment. I just wanted him inside me as soon as possible! Suddenly, he turned me around and let my nightgown fall to the floor exposing my nude body completely. "I love your body. You look amazing," he told me. A hot feeling overcame every inch of me as I melted in his hands. Bryce lifted me onto the granite counter and I accidentally tipped over the carafe full of ice cold lemonade all over my body. The coldness made my nipples even harder as he started to suck on them and push his face in between my breasts. "Mmmmm, I love your gorgeous breasts. They're so perfect. You're so perfect, Alexa. "I just smiled as he made his way down to my pussy. He opened up my thighs ever so gently and started nibbling his way to my smooth hot spot. Fuck!!! This guy is too good to be true. He knows exactly what to do. He placed his tongue on my hot clit and started to slither his way around my plump pink pussy lips. I was soaking with sweet juices that he absolutely loved to lick. "Mmmmm...baby, you taste like delicious lemonade and I just want to drink you up all night long." Bryce made me moan and groan as he continued to drive me crazy with his tongue. "I want you," I moaned to Bryce. He looked straight into my emerald green eyes, smiled and slipped his huge cock inside me and started to thrust hard. I moaned and groaned at each thrust as he went deeper and harder. He had to have been at least 9 inches long and very thick because he had my tight pussy getting hotter and wetter than ever! "Bryce, fuck me harder. I want to feel all of you inside of me. Drive me hard! Drive me crazy. Come on, baby, fuck me harder," I moaned to him louder and we both came together!

Chapter 16: The Lunch

Louisa grasped a dressing material, ventured out of the entryway of the kitchen behind the house into the chilly October daylight. She was sitting tight for the man who might before long fix the lift.

"Edward, she called! It's prepared for lunch!"

A second, she quit, tuning in, and afterward went to the grass, a little cloud went over her, and strolled over a seat, tenderly brushing the sundial with one hand as she moved by.

She was reasonably pleasant about a young lady who was little and stout, a slight lilt in her direction, and a delicate development of her hands and her legs.

"Lunch Time!" She was now able to see him, maybe at this time he was about a seventy feet away, down in the plunge on the base of the woods the kind of tall, thin man in khaki pants and dim pullover that was green, remaining adjacent to a significant blaze with a fork in his mouth, hurling thistles on to the highest point of the fire. It was thundering energetically, billows of white smoke emanating from the orange flames below. The smoke was floating over the nursery with a beautiful aroma of fall and consuming leaves. Maria went down the incline towards her dad. In the event that she wished, she may likely have made another call before she opened her eyes and allowed herself to see, however, there was something in particular about a five-star campfire that prompted her to move towards it, straight very nearby, such that she was able to feel the warmth and hear it out consume.

"Lunch," she stated, drawing closer.

"Oh, hi. Okay —yes. I'm going."

"What a decent fire."

"I've chosen to gather this spot straight up," her dad said.

"I'm wary of every one of these briers."

His gloomy look was clammy with sweat. There are little drops of it staying on his mustache like dew, and two small streams were trickling down his neck on to the turtleneck of the pullover.

"You should be cautious; you don't try too hard, Edward."

"Maria, I do wish you'd quit tending to me just as I was eighty."

"No doubt, truly, I get it. A tad of activity never hurt anyone." God, Henry! Edward! Edward! Gracious! Look! Look! Goodness! Look! Look!" The fellow turned and took a gander at Maria now, who indicated the furthest side of the fire. "That pooch! The cat!" It was a fabulous enormous feline on the planet lying close to the light, so flares frequently observed him hitting him, so he held discreetly, with his face in the sky from one viewpoint and his ears, and keeping a quiet yellow eye on his man and woman." Maria shouted, at that point she immediately dropped the treat, got it with both her arms, whisked it away, and set it on the blazes free grass.

"Your insane cat," she said, tidying off her feet.

"The spouse let me know," Cats recognize what they are doing. You won't discover a feline doing whatever they don't care for.

"Whose is it? Not felines."

"Ever before you saw it?"

"Actually, I haven't."

The feline was perched on the grass, and taking a gander at it parallel, with an inside, hidden articulation, something inquisitively omniscient and thinking and a fragile demeanor of scorn around the nose, as though seeing these two individuals, the one little, full, and ruddy, the other sweeper and sweet, was somewhat solemn.

"Be an average cat now and go on home to where you have a spot."

Her man, a significant other, started pacing around the slanted road that led to the house. The pussy cat got up and sought after, away off first, anyway edging ever closer as they came. After a short time, it was near to them; by that time, it was well in front of everyone else, similarly pacing as it asserted the entire spot, with its tail held straight open to address, like a post.

"Come all the way back," said the man. "Go on home. We needn't bother with you."

Nevertheless, at the moment when they hot home, it followed them inside, and Maria served it some warm milk inside a bowl. As everyone was enjoying their lunchtime meal, it ricocheted up to the additional seat and persevered though the lunch session with its head busy gazing at what is on the dining table.

"I couldn't care less for this cat," protested Edward.

"Goodness, I trust it's a fine catlike. I do believe it stays a brief span." Directly, listen to me, Maria. The creature can't in any capacity whatsoever stay here. It has a spot with someone else. It's lost. Moreover, if it's up 'til now endeavoring to remain close by tonight, you should take it to the police. They'll see it comes all the way back."

Immediately after Edward was don taking his lunch, he returned to his development. Maria, as anyone may have guessed, went straight to the piano. She was an experienced piano player and a real music sweetheart, and every other night, she always dedicated an hour or two of her time just to play on her own. By now, the cat was lying comfortably on the lounge chair, and as she controlled stroking it as she cruised by, the cat simply opened its eyes, looked around briefly before resuming its nap.

"You're a terribly not too bad catlike," she said. "Besides, such dazzling concealing. I wish I could keep you."

Her fingers then gently slid on top of the stairway and onto the cat's head and came across a little lump, a slight bump right over the cat's right eye.

"I feel pity for his cat," she said. "You have thumped on your first face. You ought to get old."

She walked over to the piano, sat on the long piano stool, but she was not so quick to start playing. One of her one of a kind little delights was to make a customary kind of show day, with an intentionally composed program that she figured out the detail before commencing. She was not mainly a fan of breaking pleasure by stopping while she considered what to play straightaway. All that she required was a short relief after every piece, as she was very busy gathering of onlookers hailed energetically and needed extra. It was such a lot of increasingly lovely to imagine a horde of individuals, and sometimes as she was busy playing, she was able to see an unending stockpile of chairs and what seemed to be a sea made up of white faces improved in her direction, tuning in with a bolted and admiring core interest. Occasionally, she enjoyed playing a tune or two from her memory, and sometimes she would play a song that she had overheard somewhere; that was the manner by which she felt. Moreover, what should the program be? She took a seat in front of the keyboard with her little palms got on her legs, a heavy reddening minimal individual with an around and still lovely face, she had done her hair up in an ideal bun that formed at the top of her head.

By gazing imperceptibly on to the other side, she was able to see that the cat had already settled comfortably into the love seat, and I was just amazed by the way that its dull fur lay flawlessly against the purple color of the cushion.

Shouldn't something be said about some Bach in any case? Or then again, far, and away superior, Vivaldi.

An uncommonly respectable program, one that she possessed the ability to adequately play it without the music. She edged herself nearer the piano and postponed every other time whenever a person from the group - starting at now she was able to feel like this was one of her lucky days; at the time, a person from the gathering of onlookers had just had his final hack; by then, with the moderate ease that went with about the total of her advancements, she anchored her hands up against the support and started playing. At that specific moment, she was not paying much attention to the cat, and was also unable to view the cat in any way shape or form - to be sure she had disregarded its quality - yet as the significant primary notes of the Vivaldi carefully filled the room with a melodious sound, and from the corner of a single eye, of an unexpected hurricane, a blast of improvement on the love seat on her correct side. She quit playing pronto.

"What is it?" she asked as she went to get her cat. "What's going on?"

The animal, who two or three minutes before had been resting tranquility, was directly sitting straight up on the couch, it was tense with the whole-body quivering, the ears were pointing straight up, and its eyes during the entire distance remained open, and all the time its gaze was fixated on the piano

"Did I alarm you?" she carefully asked.

"You have probably never listened to some good music before."

"No," she said, I just do not feel like it is what it is. On apprehensions, she couldn't resist touching that the cat like's mien was not one of fear. There was no contracting or venturing back. In the event that anything, there was a slanting frontward, a type of fervor regarding the animal, and the face- - well, there was to some degree an odd attitude on the front, something of a mix among stun and paralyzed.

Clearly, the substance of a cat is a slight and straight forward thing, anyway if you are observant enough to notice how the eyes and ears coordinate circumspectly, and for the most part that small area of flexible skin underneath the ears and hardly to the opposite side, you can at times watch the impression of inconceivable sentiments. Maria was watching the face eagerly now, and in light of the fact that she was quite intrigued to witness what will happen in the ensuing time, she associated her hands to the reassurance and started playing the Vivaldi.

Exercise

Emotions in Motion

TIME TO READ: 3 MINUTES

TIME TO DO: 7 MINUTES

Emotions come from our mood, circumstances, and relationships with others. We label these feelings as good or bad. One technique for managing emotions is to acknowledge them and shift them in the opposite direction. Research has shown that smiling—even when we feel down—can help our body produce serotonin and dopamine, the happy hormones.

No matter how you feel emotionally, use this exercise to shift your feelings because—this is important to remember—emotions are about how you feel about something and you can easily control them using exercises like this one. This exercise will use 2 + 4 breathing.

1. Close your eyes and take a moment to note your emotions.

2. While doing 2 + 4 breathing, notice where in your body the emotion is located and place your hands over that area.
3. Smile and say to yourself or out loud, "I choose happiness." Repeat the phrase.
4. While doing 2 + 4 breathing again, smile and open your eyes. Notice the shift in your emotions. Repeat the phrase 10 times.

Chapter 17: The Older Adult

The older adult heard a far-off thundering and turned his eyes to the sky. He was seeking a gravely required downpour to guarantee a full collection. "A cloudless sky," he murmured. Out there, he thought he saw a herd of dark flying creatures flying in an exceptional example. At that point, he saw men running rapidly from the fields yelling, "It is the Japanese!" The ranchers would be the fortunate ones today. The individuals who lived in the city were most certainly not.

The Japanese aviators took an enjoyment watching individuals on the ground dispersing like mice. They snickered and yelled "Banzai" to one another. Executing was such a simple errand against such an unprotected populace.

Before long there would be no resistance to Japan's requirement for painfully required assets. The Emperor required nourishment for his kin, work for his industry, and oil to keep up Japan's military mastery.

The Far East would turn out to be a piece of his Empire. The Chinese, they guaranteed, ought to be thankful for their new sovereign … all things considered, they were "freeing" the Chinese from the "remote fallen angels."

Their celebration was hindered by the shouting sound of planes originating from above. The rear turret heavy armament specialist's eyes enlarged in dread at seeing a warplane with the substance of a fearsome tiger shark painted on its nose.

"Flying Tigers!" the kids yelled, while the grown-ups pulled them to security. When resistance to those "noxious dwarves" from Japan appeared to be vain, it was seeing these bold American pilots that were viewed as a blessing from their divine beings. Each time one of the aircrafts was taken out of the sky in a wad of fire or seen diving to the earth, there was an extraordinary cheering from the workers.

One of the pilots accompanying one of the Mitsubishi Ki-21 "Sally" overwhelming aircraft, named "Sally's" by the Americans, got maddened by his powerlessness to get the escaping tigers and looked for retaliation by strafing a gathering of youngsters who had walked out reasoning that the threat had passed. They could see the pilot chuckling as the slugs tore through the little one's bodies sending them flying into the air like cloth dolls.

"That son of bitch!" yelled Ricky Caruso, one of the "Tigers" who had seen the slaughter. He put his nose into a lofty jump and started to pound the Ki-27 with slugs from his .50-gauge nose weapons. The pilot zigged and zoomed Caruso's P-40 War hawk's unrivaled speed yet in a plunge found the "Nate," and inside seconds, the plane was ablaze. He could see the Japanese pilot squirming miserably as the blazes devoured his substance.

'Consume in Hell, you charlatan!' Ricky's idea as he pulled up from his plunge.

"Post Rico!" a yell came over the radio. "You have a Jap on your tail!" Ricky went to look when he saw slugs tear into his conservative. He dunked his wing and went into a shallow jump wanting to evade his assailant.

"Try not to attempt to battle him, Rico! That little dark-colored jerk's unreasonably agile for you. I'm coming, simply keep him off of your tail."

Ricky zigged and crossed; however, the Japanese pilot was resolved to get his retribution. 'I figure I may have gotten it this time,' he thought. He felt a crash hit the rear of his seat secured by a thick defensive layer plate and realized that the following slug might discover him.

Out of nowhere, he heard one of the Tigers plunging and saw tracer projectiles flying past him. He saw the Jap contender, another Nakajima Ki-43, or "Oscar" as the Americans alluded to it, fly away with a severely harmed tail fold. There was yelling over the radio, and things like: "Go get that jerk," and "make him meet his progenitors," yet the Tiger let him go and reacted in an unmistakable and quiet Midwestern drawl: "I'll get him next time."

Ricky perceived the voice. It was his best and dearest companion, Lars "Bull" Lundgren, the stumbling ranch kid from Minnesota. He heard the thunder of a motor to one side and saw Ox's whole toothed smile gazing back at him.

"I owe you one!" Ricky snickered, yet the trial had obviously shaken him.

Volunteers

The one thing you learn in the military is never to chip in, or so the platitude goes, yet the children of the Great Depression knew whenever there was a chance to be had, you needed to bounce on it. Ricky and Ox were two of those children.

Ricky and Ox were the two most improbable companions that one could envision. Ricky was a wiry minimal Italian-American child from New Jersey with a smart mouth and a belligerent disposition. The bull was a rancher's child from America's heartland... a blundering monster of Swedish stock, calm, with a quiet aura that gave a false representation of his high astuteness. The two of them made them thing in like manner. They were acceptable with anything mechanical and wanted to fly.

There was a genuine push by the American Government to reinforce its air corps. During the middle of the Depression, Hollywood turned out movies that celebrated pilots as legends, confronting peril in the skies. They longed for turning out to be Aces, that is, to score at any rate five executes against the adversary. Why stop at five. Most likely, the Red Baron's score of eighty must be outperformed? Wasn't America the best nation on the planet?

The war in China had been continuing for very nearly ten years when they get for Volunteers turned out in March of 1941. The Russians had been helping the Chinese battle the Japanese, yet now was pulling out and making a beeline to meet the more noteworthy risk from Hitler. The German war machine was traveling through Poland and smashing the entirety of the Soviet protections.

Chiang Kai-Shek, the pioneer of the Nationalists in China, approached the American Government, on edge that Japan's authority in Asia would go unchecked, for help. Ricky and Ox thought nothing about China, yet they realized that a war was approaching between Imperial Japan and the United States.

"We got to get right now they come here!" was the catchphrase heard everywhere throughout the airbases the nation over. The pilots were all the while flying the old biplanes and were kicking the bucket to get their hands on the new Curtiss P-40's.

Ricky and Ox met in flight school. They alternated being the tops in their group, however, Ricky pushed out Ox in the aeronautical battle moves and didn't let him overlook it.

"Hello, Ox!" Ricky cried. "Com'ere, take a gander at this."

Bull, who was never one to be excessively energized, gradually strolled over to his companion who was on his toes attempting to peruse the note that some insightful ass nailed high to the release board.

"Put me down, douche bag!" Ricky reprimanded as he wriggled out of the large man's hold.

"I didn't see a stepping stool 'round here so I figured you might require a lift" Ox giggled.

"Tune in up Ox. It says here that they need fliers in China. Volunteers will be released from the equipped administrations, to be utilized for "preparing and guidance" by a private military contractual worker, the Central Aircraft Manufacturing Company (CAMCO). They'll pay $600 every month for pilot officials, $675 per month for flight pioneers, $750 for squadron pioneers and about $250 for talented ground crew members. A portion of the folks said that they would get 500 bucks for each Jap that they destroy!"

"I don't know, and you need to leave the Army to join. Is it accurate to say that you are certain you need to change it for an undertaking?"

"Listen to Ox. On the off chance that we get over yonder and kill a few Japs and become Aces, at that point we could bring in some decent cash, return with fight understanding, and re-enroll. We can't lose... except if... you're a major chicken?"

"They call me Ox, not chicken. Alright, little man, I'm in!"

That mid-year, Ox, Ricky, and around 100 other "volunteers'" boarded ships bound for Burma conveying regular citizen visas. They were at first based at a British runway in Tango for preparing while their airplane was amassed and test flown by CAMCO staff at Mingaladon Airport, only outside of Rangoon. General Chennault, the establishing pioneer of the American Volunteer Group, set up a school building that was made fundamental because numerous pilots had "lied about their flying experience, guaranteeing interest experience when they had flown just aircraft and once in a while considerably less ground-breaking planes.

It wasn't some time before each man had his image spankings' new P-40 War hawks that the Brits turned down as out of date. They would confront the Japanese warrior, the Nakajima Ki-27, a slower, yet progressively agile contender in the hands of an accomplished flier. Chennault cautioned them not to be maneuvered into a dogfight. On the off chance that they had to draw in, the men were advised to place their plane into a lofty jump and pull up quickly. Any Japanese pilot sufficiently silly to attempt to get them would separate in mid-air as they couldn't deal with the "G" powers in their delicate manufactured airplane.

Aircraft were focused on. P-40 pilots were told to swoop down like winged animals of prey from high heights and lay into the plane squadrons with overpowering firepower. "Hit them rigid," and get the damnation out of there!

"Presently it's close to home!"

Ricky and Ox were working off a headache when the news came:

"Hello Guys, get your butts out of bed! Fitz shouted. The Colonel needs everyone out as soon as possible. We got great news from Pearl Harbor!"

"I feel like poo!" Ricky groaned.

"You look like poo!" Ox giggled.

"You'll be in poop on the off chance that you don't get your rear ends up brisk" cautioned Fitz.

There was protesting among the youngsters as they bobbled on that early December morning. They sat in the field house hanging tight for the Colonel.

Exercise

Calm Breaths

TIME TO READ: 3 MINUTES

TIME TO DO: 7 MINUTES

Do you have a potentially stressful situation coming up? Maybe you have a big history test, or you had a fight with a friend and are worried about seeing them in school. Don't worry—this exercise will help you gain confidence and calm with mindful breathing.

1. In a quiet room, sit comfortably in a chair with your feet placed firmly on the ground. Gently rest your hands on your stomach. Set a timer for 7 minutes; use your phone if you don't have a timer handy.

2. Close your eyes and focus on your breathing. Breathe slowly until you can move the breath down to your belly. Place your hands on your stomach and feel it gently rise and fall.

3. While doing the 4, 7, 8 breathing (Yoga Breath), say to yourself or out loud, "I can confidently take care of my day." Repeat three times.

4. Return to breathing normally, with eyes closed, until the timer completes.

Chapter 18: The Time Travel

In the fabric of space and time, there is woven a passage that allows for travel between. The realms were not knit as a waterproof cloak. There are seams and streams that beings can slip between. A displacement of creatures in the wrong time or a displacement of matter in the wrong space is a hint at this "Stairway between Realms." It has been used by the bold and brave to pass to new dimensions and discover new secrets. Many geniuses have wielded this power to expand their minds. But there is a danger there.

If you travel for too long along the Stairway Between Realms, you may lose your way. The passage is not clear as a hallway or a literal stream. It was a convoluted maze that intertwines and intersects upon itself. Imagine an ouroboros that was eating its own tail, but twisting and knotting itself as it did so. This is what the Stairway between Realms can be like. So if you take this leap, be careful. You may not be able to leap back.

The other danger lies in the door itself. You may be able to enter. You may be able to exit. Perhaps you can even exit when and where you wish. But that does not mean you are the only one. There are other beings out there that can do the same. And some of them are purely interdimensional beings that dwell purely in between realms. Watch yourself as you travel along the Stairway between Realms. Protect yourself. But more importantly, protect time and space itself. If you risk releasing one of these beings out into your dimension or another, be responsible. Find another route.

There was once a man named Leonard How lite. He was a dimensional passenger who rode for most of his life on the Stairway between Realms. He fancied himself quite the expert. But Leonard How lite had passed along the Stairway between Realms all of ten to twenty times. He'd seen thirty-five realms, despite only using the passage between them twenty times. Still, for all his knowledge of the passage and the few places he had traveled to, he did not have the sense to take precautions. For example, he never disguised himself or masked his identity. If he traveled to the future or past, he wore his own features like a mask. He thought that if he was not in his own dimension, there was no fear.

Wrong! Leonard How lite met many versions of himself on his trip through the Stairway between Realms? And upon meeting himself, he created a paradox in that dimension that sent its native Leonard How lite into a pocket. The pockets would hold that Leonard there until the paradox untangled itself. Of course, this really bummed Leonard How lite out. He had gone back at one point to help himself out. Not possible, it seemed.

Another troublesome situation also burst out of the Stairway between Realms thanks to Leonard How lite. You see, he passed between the dimensions with relative ease, but believed he was all alone in that passage. Of course, he was wrong. The shifters, beings that shift between dimensions, stalked Leonard How lite through the passage and were set loose upon several dimensions. Learning this, Leonard did go back and salvage what he could. Most of those universes were already lost, however.

Now, to be fair to Leonard, he's saved the multiverse several times. On multiple occasions, he's undone someone else's dimensional catastrophe. He's untangled paradox for other folks, slew many shifters, and unjumbled the space-time stream in general. He's also trained many individuals on proper Stairway between Realms protocol. So remember, you can be like Leonard How lite. Or you can be like Leonard How lite. Your choice!

Exercise

What's Your Name?

Exercise time: 10 minutes

Benefits: Fosters expression and increases self-esteem

MATERIALS: Assorted markers, 1 sheet of 18-by-24-inch heavy-weight drawing paper

1. Using block letters, write your name in any color on your paper from left to right.
2. Think of a positive word that has the same first letter as your name. Add this word to your drawing in any location on the paper.
3. Pick your favorite colors and create a design inside the letters of your name

Chapter 19: A Bargain

Magda hadn't considered the weather reports when she made her way into the woods that day. The weather had been sunny, and the temperatures had been rather mild all week long. **Why should that suddenly change just because I've got errands to do outside?** She wondered to herself as she grumbled about the rain clouds that were rolling in overhead.

As the clouds muddied the blue sky above, Magda remained determined to complete the tasks that had sent her out to the woods. She would get the photo she needed for her photography class. Marlon had told her not to bother taking the photography class, as he deemed it a waste of money. He said that Magda never finished anything she ever set herself to and that there wasn't any reason to expect that this endeavor of becoming a photographer to be any different than her failed ventures into pottery, woodworking, painting, and macramé.

Out of spite, Magda signed up for the classes, which had begun in August of that year. She had attended every single class, completed every single assignment, gone above and beyond to learn more about it in her spare time, and had shown Marlon that she meant to prove him wrong on this one. Marlon, of course, didn't care about it one way or the other. He just wanted Magda to find something that would fill her time and make her happy. If that thing happened to be taking photos just to spite him, he figured that worked just well enough.

As Magda got deeper into the woods, the trees seemed to drink in every bit of light that streamed in from the sky, leaving very little for the forest floor below. In spite of the terrible conditions this created for photography, and in spite of Magda's comprehensive understanding of how lighting worked, she pressed on, looking for the perfect scene to shoot. She had seen it days before but hadn't had her camera with her. She told herself that she had only been scouting and that there was no need to bring her camera with her. In retrospect, she realized that she should have brought the camera so she could capture that moment.

She had found a small, unique grouping of mushrooms in the forest that had a unique, seemingly purposeful formation among them. They were arranged in a perfect circle and the odds of this, Magda thought, were slim to none! She had to get her camera and come back for a photo. For all she knew now, however, deer or other woodland creatures had come by and eaten the mushrooms. For all she knew, they could have been trampled by an unknowing moose traveling through the wood. Still, she pressed onward to the area where she had remembered seeing them.

As she approached the area where she had remembered seeing them just a couple of days previously, she held her breath. She wasn't sure how she would react if they were no longer in the place where she had last seen them, but she knew that Marlon would see the brunt of her anger about the situation. He wouldn't have really been to blame for whatever had eaten or trampled them, nor would he be to blame for her neglecting to bring her camera when she had come scouting earlier in the week. He would, however, be responsible for getting under her skin, but that was a badge of honor she knew he would proudly wear. For that, she would hold this whole ordeal against him until he soothed her with forehead kisses and hot chocolate.

She crested a small mound in the woods and breathed a sigh of relief. The mushrooms were still there, and they looked as fresh and bright as they had when she came to scout. There was something alluring about those mushrooms and the formation in which they grew. She snapped her shot and marveled at how perfectly her camera captured their likeness. She failed to remember the looming clouds overhead and that there should not have been ample light in these woods to so beautifully capture the mushrooms in that way. She saw nothing odd about the light that flowed seemingly from nowhere to illuminate her shot.

"Beautiful shot," a delicate voice came from the branch above her head. Magda's head shot up to find a rather diminutive woman sitting on the branch.

"Oh, thank you. I'm sorry, I didn't see you there before."

"I didn't mean to startle you. May I see your shot?" Magda slowly held the camera out to the woman in the tree. It wasn't until Magda's camera was in the woman's hands that Magda realized how impossibly tiny this woman really was. The camera sat in her lap in much the same way that a child might hold a gentleman's briefcase. The woman commented on the composition of her shot, the lighting, and the angle.

"You really know your stuff, Magda. Great work. I'm sure Mr. Yamashida will be impressed with it." Magda's blood ran cold. How could this impossibly tiny woman know her name, the name of her photography instructor, or that this shot was for an assignment? The trepidation and alarm must have been plain on Magda's face.

"You're not as quiet as you think, wandering through these woods. All I had to do was listen for about five minutes before I felt like I was a part of your world." Magda heaved a sigh.

"Oh, man. I didn't even realize I was talking. I'm so sorry." She chuckled at herself, taking the camera back from the woman and setting about returning the device to its carrying case.

"I'm Saoirse, by the way."

"It's nice to meet you, S... Saoi—"
"Saoirse. It's okay, it's an Irish Gaelic name that's hard to pronounce." Magda nodded, a little embarrassed.

"So, do you spend a lot of time in trees?" Saoirse giggled to herself.

"You could say that I do, yeah. Do you spend a lot of time cursing in the woods?"

"You could say that I do, yeah." Magda and Saoirse laughed. "I like to scout for photo locations in places where nature is more present than man. I find that I capture the best photos in locations like that."

"Ah, yes. Nature has a lot of beauty to offer, indeed."

"I'm so grateful I got here when I did," Magda said, looking down at the mushrooms. "The light is so dim here now. I wouldn't have been able to get nearly as good a shot in this light."

"I thought that might be the case. I added a little more lighting from up here when you were lining up your shot. I didn't want you to have to hold today against... Marlon, was it?" Magda laughed again at her unwitting oversharing.

"Yes, Marlon it was. Thank you for that. What did you use?" Magda looked around but saw no equipment.

"Oh, a little of this, a little of that. My question is, what would you give me in return for that perfect shot?" Saoirse kept a cool smirk on her face as she maintained eye contact with Magda, who froze. She hadn't expected to end up in debt to someone she didn't know, for a favor she didn't ask them to do for her.

"I'm not sure... What did you have in mind?"

"Well, I was wondering if you might help me find my way back out of the woods? I'm quite small, as you can see, and I'm a little bit worried something might nip me by the scruff and carry me off." Magda raised her eyebrows.

"Oh, certainly. I can show you out. Do you need a ride to the main road?"

"You know, that would be lovely. Help me out of this tree, would you love?" Saoirse lifted her arms so Magda could take hold of her like a small child. As Magda guided her safely to the ground, she marveled at the size of this woman. She really was the size of an infant, with the proportions of a woman. It was baffling. **Perhaps some form of dwarfism with very little proportion disparity,** she thought.

Just as Saoirse's feet hit the ground, she took hold of Magda's wrists and began speaking a language Magda didn't understand. Immediately. Magda's knees buckled and she was crouched in the center of the circle, arms outstretched and held in place by the tiny creature. Saoirse's eyes glowed as she spoke English once again.

"It's nothing personal, Magda. I just needed a way out and you were in the right place at the right time." Magda felt her very essence sliding out of her body. It seemed nearly like a phantom limb phenomenon when she swore that she could feel Saoirse's essence seeping into her body where hers had just been. Suddenly, the world seemed massive.

Magda's body stood up before her, looking at her hands, breathing in deeply and making strange motions with her hands.

"No magic. I'm free." Saoirse, now in Magda's body, looked down at Magda. "Thank you. I know you will hate me for this, but please know that you have my sincerest, undying gratitude." At this, she grabbed the camera bag and ran out of the woods toward Magda's car.

Magda, now in Saoirse's tiny body, ran as quickly as she could to keep up with the body that had just been stolen from her.

"Wait! Come back!" She was still yards away when the car rumbled to life and lurched as the driver tried to figure out how to make it work. She kept running, feeling the burning in her lungs as she did so.

Just as she reached the road where her car was parked, it was as though she slammed into a thick pane of unyielding glass with full force. She bounced off the barrier and fall onto her bottom. Her car sped off, leaving her in these woods forever.

Magda had never meant to trade her whole life for the perfect shot.

Chapter 20: The Super Star

I was born in Philadelphia, or Philly, as some locals like to call it. I have always been a hyperactive kid since infancy. Mother would always gleefully describe how I never woke up grumpy and how I always greeted each new day with a smile and how I rarely ever cried, even as a baby. How I got to walk just before I was 10-months old and how I loved throwing and kicking virtually anything around once my arms and feet could carry them. I seem to have been born with more energy than your average kid.

I used to think my family is the best there is, maybe not as much as when I was a kid, but somewhere in my heart, I still feel so. My Dad's a salesman, a hardworking and diligent one. On most days, he would leave the house very early and return late in the evening. And even when he was home, he would spend so many hours on the phone making series of deliberations that rarely resulted in money. Well, not enough money to get me a PlayStation4 like the other kids on the block. My mother used to work as a janitor back in Philly, but after my dad's employers transferred him to Washington, DC, mum stayed unemployed for a while before working as a sales attendant in a superstore.

From a young age, I always loved adventure. Back in Philly, I loved to take really slow walks to school and sniff in the scent of the air, the air seemed to have this musty, inexplicable smell of history. One that I loved to feel as the cool morning breeze blew against my face, this is still what I miss the most about Philly. More than my friends, more than my school. Can't say I miss it more than those occasional cheesesteaks dad got us though. I really didn't have many friends back in my elementary school days, I always loved to speed back home after school. I had no time for the characteristic slow walks that most friends, or group of friends, had after school. I'd run home to watch the older boys play basketball in the mega court that overlooked our house. Whenever I could muster the calmness, I loved to seat on the benches outside the main court and watch them through the netted gauze as my headphones blared some hip-hop.

Other times, I just stood and watched, then practice when they leave. My sister, Alissa, never seemed to understand why we were so different. Why I'd rather walk slowly in the mornings while she's in a haste and runs home in the afternoons when she's more relaxed and strolling with her few friends. Compared to me, she's the rather somber and taciturn one and would rather stay indoors, solve arithmetic and read literature.

On arrival to DC, life, in general, seemed to get a little better – or was it the improved environment that made it seem so? – Dad got a pay raise at work and mum got a better job two months later, anything's better than being a janitor. Our new school was way better, there was no need for taking slow or fast walks to and from school. We joined our peers on the school bus daily. I can still recall my first day on the bus, I hopped on feeling like the coolest kid on the block, but these DC kids seem to be mad at me for being so cool.

None of them would make space for me to the seat, each chair I found some space and attempted to seat what I heard the kids say was, "Taken!". For at least the first five rows, all I heard was "Taken!", I was beginning to think this word meant something to these DC folks and was also contemplating putting up a fight with a rather feeble-looking guy who somehow managed to look more troublesome than every other kid on the bus. And till he relocated with his parents to Wichita, I still considered him the most troublesome kid in the school.

My thoughts of landing a punch on Allan's face was cut short by Derek, he beckoned on me from the back to come to share his seat. I remember pausing for a while to observe the little-big guy, he had bright blue eyes and dirty blond hair. He did seem a little taller than most other kids, but had this aura of happiness around him. A jolly good fellow, Derek Jones.

I bonded with Derek really quickly and along several lines. We both arrived DC recently, he arrived only a week before me. His dad had also been transferred from Pennsylvania State, but not from my Philly, they had lived in Pittsburgh, and many other cities, his Dad's job is quite nomadic. Derek also had my dream PlayStation4 and his parents would let me sleepover so we stay up and play some of the coolest video games till his mum comes into his room to shut off the power and ask us to sleep. On one of those really crazy nights, we still played more games after she left, we just readjusted the curtains and turned down the volume to it's barest minimum, but what connected me and Derek the most was our love for sports.

Although we spent hours talking about the most popular sports like baseball and football, it was basketball that took most of our talk-time. We would often sit and talk about basketball for hours on end arguing from the better basketball team between the Philadelphia 76ers and the Washington Wizards to the better player between Michael Jordan and LeBron James. Basketball, our one true love. And we'd always talk about how dreamt of being renowned jocks in high school and how we aspired to make it to the NBA and surpass the feats achieved by Michael Jordan.

At age 9, I and Derek saved up some money from the little stipends offered us by our parents to get snacks during class breaks. Just enough money to get a basketball. Oh, how we loved it! It was our biggest achievement and the most valuable asset at the time. We'd practice bouncing and dribbling on a tiled slab in the courtyard behind Derek's family house. Derek's mum, a school teacher renowned for her strictness with kids, would always shout and warn whenever she began to hear the incessant sound of our ball thumping against the floor, "Hey you boys, do remember that's no basketball court and play carefully enough to avoid breaking the window louvres or the car windscreen", she'd say as though it were some over-rehearsed line for a school play.

We even became so conversant with the warnings that we'd recite them alongside. We thought we had it all figured out and that we could avoid breakages and similar accidents, after all, we've been doing so for almost a year of playing. Then one day, we got so engrossed in the game with burning passion to emulate our idols, Michael Jordan and LeBron James, we thought to try a slam dunk and smash the ball against a small round circle we had marked on the wall and we were doing just great. It was in that moment of euphoria that I picked up the ball, jumped as high as my legs could carry and struck it against the wall with more force than I ever thought I could muster. Impressive, aye? But the ball bounced off the wall with a widely different angle and struck Mrs. Jones' car.

With our hearts in our mouths, we ran towards the car to examine the degree of damage done, deep down I was hoping there was no damage done, but my hopes were shattered this time, although the side mirror was much more shattered. It was while we were still examining the damage done that I felt a firm grip behind me, right on my waist and I was being pulled backwards, I could also see Derek involuntarily moving backwards. Apparently, Mrs. Jones had heard the sound and was standing behind us all the while till she decided to pull us in to mete out whatever punishment she deemed fit for these two moderately-insolent, excessively passionate and young basketballers.

We got the scolding of our lives especially because Derek and I both claimed responsibility for the accident. I was the culprit, but he took it upon himself, the good lad he is. Derek was grounded every day after school for a whole week, even his video game console was confiscated. Tough times. The occurrence marked the end of our basketball escapades in the Jones' family compound. We had to look elsewhere.

After Derek's dark days of ostracism, we had to sit down and re-strategize, we weren't about to contemplate shunning our dreams. Our dreams of being highly envied high school jocks. Our dreams of getting a sports scholarship to college and eventually making it to the NBA and surpassing the feats achieved by Michael Jordan and LeBron James. Big dreams for little guys, but we've always been so imaginative. We still spent hours talking, just talking.

More of basketball, but soon new names outside basketball started popping up in our conversations, names like Tricia and Angela, or Angie, as Derek liked to call her, but that wasn't until we turned 12 and started middle school. For now, we resorted to trying out for the school junior team and visiting the basketball court in the area to watch the older boys play. Once in a while they'd let us play with them, maybe as a result of a shortage of players or just to show us some love. The first few occasions we got to bounce a ball with the big guys, we goofed. I was really tensed up and the urge to impress somehow made me shiver.

Although I was already growing taller than most kids my age, I felt quite infinitesimal in their midst and would often give the ball away faster than I got the ball. Derek was even playing better than me – so I thought, though he'd often say he felt I played better – We soon experienced great improvement though and when it was time for the school junior team tryouts, it didn't take so much effort for us to get picked. Coach Bradley Grant would often say we're the future of the game and if we keep working hard, we'll someday lead our high school senior team to national glory and land ourselves scholarships. He loved to say this whenever he met just the two of us training, he'd never say it to the hearing of the other boys. Maybe he doesn't want to make them feel less. Or maybe he just says just about the same thing to every kid on the team to boost their morale, but that would mean we're not exceptional. I still think I and Derek are the best players in the team though, after all, we're the only three-point specialists on the team.

Our basketball skills at such a young age brought us a lot of attention. Once upon a time, all the kids said "Taken!" when I hopped on the bus, but nowadays virtually every kid wants to seat with me on the bus and in the class. My grades didn't suffer, mama always says "The best athletes also took their studies seriously", "Michael Jordan is a college graduate", she'd say. These motivated me to study and make good grades too.

Although I've never been great at math and arithmetic, but Alissa who could pass as a genius would always help. At least until Tricia came into the picture. Tricia was the best student in the class, beautiful and quite shy. Sometimes during classes, I steal glances at her. Sometimes I feel she steals glances at me too, but it's probably because I stare too much. We started spending some time together during breaks and she'd put me through some math I found complex, most times I caught myself thinking about her rather than listening to her though, but nevertheless, I preferred her tutelage to my sister. I just loved listening to her speak. I think I began to like her in some funny kind of way as we see in movies, but in movies, such feelings usually involve teens and adults and I'm just a 12-year old junior high school kid. I got to mention it to Derek, "I think I like Tricia", I said shyly hoping he won't burst into loud laughter and make me feel worse. He assumed a straight, emotionless face before he burst out the words "I think I like Angie", he said in a somewhat hushed tone.

Apparently, he had been experiencing something similar, but felt odd about it and was too shy to talk about it, even to me. We decided to just move on with it since we were both in it then it was probably normal. Although we still have their names popping up in our conversations every now and then.

By this time we were already in 8th grade and middle school was drawing to an end. Anticipating freshman year at the Montgomery County Public Schools. My dreams are as high as ever for my basketball and my academic career. Mama says asides being exceptional in my game, good grades can boost my chances of getting a scholarship. High school would be fun with basketball, just one thing can go wrong. Derek! Derek's dad has been transferred to Madison, Wisconsin.

When we spoke this morning, he said his mum is still contemplating quitting her job and relocating the entire family. For now, we don't know if he'll be leaving. I honestly hope he doesn't. I'll miss him, he's been there since my day one in DC and we've done literally everything together. High school would be fun and all, but much less without my buddy. Something in me still hopes he'll stay back in DC for whatever reason.

I'll turn fourteen tomorrow and I'll be starting high school next week, I just decided to take out some time to reminisce some key points of my life and dream my dreams. The future lies before me like paths of pure white snow, I'll tread carefully because every step will show. Stay tuned and watch out for the next Michael Jordan.

Chapter 21: A Hike in the Forest

Before we begin this journey downwards into the deepest realms of our subconscious, let us take a minute to physically and mentally and spiritually acclimate ourselves into being with awareness of our inner-sanctum, our internal workings. We will begin by going to a place of comfort, ideally a bed, or a very comfortable reclining chair, and we will relax our bodies to the furthest extent possible. Now, close your eyes, staying firmly on your back, with your arms relaxed at your sides and your legs rested downwards. Take one deep breath in, through your nostrils, counting slowly to four, and one deep breath out, through your nostrils again, counting slowly to four. Breathe in the breath of the spirit and breathe out the stress of the day. Now is the time to rest. Become aware of nothing but the air flowing through your nostrils, envision a steady flowing stream, smooth inhalations and exhalations, your body become weightier and more relaxed with each passing cycle of breath. Allow your thoughts to become completely still, as you focus on your core, your solar plexus, allowing your thoughts to flow outwards past your vision until they escape your being, while only holding and retaining the pure awareness of spirit, the holy serenity of the mind and body. Breathe in, one, two, three, four, then breathe out, one, two, three, four, each breath becoming slower. One... two... three... four... One... two... three... four... One... two... three... four... One... two... three... four... One... two... three... four... One... two... three... four... Continue this pattern of breath, expanding, and sink down deeper into yourself, becoming a voyeur of your own still, relaxed body, lost in time. Become lost in this experience as you journey further into the trance, and prepare for the road we are about to embark upon. Draw further and further away from your still, lying body, and into the realm of imagination, where images grow, the land of dreams that you are about to become one with. Erase your mind of all that is within it currently, and prepare the landscape for a new and fresh experience, in the farther reaches of reality. One... two... three... four... inhale... One... two... three... four... exhale... One... two... three... four... inhale... One... two... three... four... exhale... Now, with your mind, body, and spirit rested totally, entranced, and fertile, let us begin.

You had overheard someone at a local café talking about a strange and secluded place less than an hour up into the mountains that is relatively untouched by man, a slight miracle, and totally accessible. You have the day off, so you decide to go and see it for yourself. The drive there is strangely serene. This must be a day that a lot of people decided to stay indoors, because there is almost no traffic on the roads, becoming less and less as you go further up the mountain roads. The weather is just right, not too hot and just a little bit cool. You decide not to listen to any music on your trip, as you feel it would only distract you from yourself, and you feel very comfortable with yourself right now. Outside your car windows, the density of the trees increases, making it harder and harder to recognize where one tree begins and the other ends. Eventually, you are in a sea of green, bleeding into an infinite blue sea above it. You begin to feel totally grounded yet totally enlightened, your feet on the ground yet your head in the clouds. You've forgotten that you are even driving by the time you get to your destination. You step out of your car and you feel like you've been there all along. The trailhead is incredibly esoteric, yet totally and naturally definite, as if the trees have made their own way just for you to progress. You don't even remember what it was that signified to you that this is where you were heading, no sign that you recall having seen, yet you took just the right turn and ended up exactly where you wanted to be. A couple of feet further down the way, and your car disappears from your sight, and you are totally entrenched in a brown and green void that you seem to be directly in the middle of. The tops of the trees seem to make a sky in their own right, and the blue sky above them seems to be a more ethereal divine abyss beyond this. Immediately, wildlife begins to bristle all around you. Each tree, and there are thousands, spread infinitely, is alive, it seems, with it's own colony of critters, scurrying up and down the shafts of the trees where they blend into the vast array of birds fluttering to and fro across each tree top. Deer cross your path without a second thought, as if you are nothing to them but another tree among the infinite. You do not disrupt them. Each and every green patch among the endless dirt is bristling, and you know that each one houses its own infinite array of life, from the visible to the microscopic. Each speck of dirty is alive with more life than you can possibly see. The sounds of all this life together form a grand orchestral score, with the percussion of the breeze against the limbs of the trees and the greenery being it's ephemeral skeleton. There are the violas and violins of the chirping birds making their own independent songs, and the soft and expressive squeaks of the chipmunks and squirrels and smaller things tied to the ground. There are the cellos of the four-legged herbivores, close and off in the distance, communicating to each other in a language you cannot understand literally but feel a close relationship to in some way intangible to your own waking experience. And, off in the distance, there are the bass growls of the grand beasts that hide in the shadows, far away from you, giving you your space as you give them theirs. All the while, your footsteps against the grass and the dirt and the leaves and the twigs form their own accouterment to this vast symphony, a tiny little dance in a great and grand field, tying everything together. You stop for a second and hold your hands out, and into your palms form a connective embrace with this infinite multitude of life before and behind and above you. All this, you are a part of, as it is a part of you, the natural order of things, the earth and the sky and the dirt and below. Above and below, the life that expands infinitely outwards. You feel totally whole in this vast open nature, and for a moment you just stand in its existence, a part of it. Then you move on. Further and further down the trail, the wilderness growing denser and denser as the tree tops close in on the skies above them, the light become scanter and scanter as if to pay its respects to the exponentially growing depths of this wide-spreading forest. Eventually, you are no longer sure if it is night or day, but everything is awake, and you can see it all. The earth glows and radiates into you with ancient and uncompromising power. You cannot believe that before, in this same day, you were among men in their cities, at the café, overhearing about this strange and magical place. Somehow, these two worlds exist as one. Yet you are here, now, and feel as if you always have been, and as if the world of the city had never really existed. There was only this, just you, and this infinite nature at your fingertips, and you at its. In the close distance there is a glowing light, and you begin to hear the sounds of rushing water growing stronger and stronger. This sound and sight is accompanied by a cool, moist feeling in the air, as if an ancient spirit is welcoming you into its embrace, and you are being swallowed by its presence as if into the belly of a great whale. This entrance becomes closer and closer, and you feel yourself being overtaken by the golden light emanating so thoroughly defined through this infinite abyss of dark, deep wilderness you have found yourself in the midst of. You slowly but surely make your way, as the sound of the water becomes almost all there is, drowning out so beautifully the choir of the mountains, as you transcend that golden light and find yourself in the valley of a great and roaring river, starting from one eternity and going into the next, farther and farther each way then the eye could ever see. It is day; there can be no doubt, and the brightest, purest day you could ever imagine. The sky is the bluest it has ever been; as if all the air that has ever existed has parted its way for you to totally connect to the sun, straight through the atmosphere. The sight and the sound totally overtakes you, and you feel for a moment as if you are a planet unto yourself, hurtling at the speed of light through space, yet totally and serenely still, and totally alone yet loved in the abyss of the universe. You realize, here, now, it is your time to rest. You sit down, and for a long time, maybe years, you stare at the river rushing forward through time, on and on, forever. Nighttime comes, and goes, and comes, and goes, and the river never stops. You feel as if you have entered an eternal hibernation, having totally melded your consciousness with the vast and flowing river, and the infinite wilderness that adorns it from every direction, no longer needing any independent being or state of awareness. You are there for as long as the earth itself has existed, and will. Behind you, a series of clomps awaken you. It is a great and grand beast of the forest, standing tall as the trees, with antlers that seem to scratch the heavens. He sits down beside you, lying next to you, and rests with you. You realize there are others, besides you, others existing just as close to you in this infinite wilderness as this. You lazily doze off together, and fall into his great coat, feeling his breathing, which seems to be the rumble of the entire earth, forever, and you fall asleep.

Chapter 22: The Train Journey

You listen to the passengers on the train as they whisper amongst one another.

They all seem to be on their way to very important places.

Watching humanity from the outside always lends to the idea that everyone is on a mission, except for you.

Little do any of them know, that is the point of this day for you.

You have been so busy with your work and so stressed about your bills, that today your only goal is to escape the grind.

You're going to find a place of stillness and peace.

The steady roar of the train wheels is already relaxing you.
You watch your chest rising and falling slowly as the noises around you fade into one sound.

Your head falls back against your headrest as you watch the scenery from the windows.

Fields of pale green grass roll past your eyes, broken up only by the occasional cow.

The sky above is a perfect baby blue with fluffy clouds of cotton that tower into the atmosphere.

You could not have asked for better weather for your adventure.

Slowly the world outside begins to shift.

You are still tuned into the constant noise of the train, but your view from the window is becoming more interesting.

A few picturesque barns have whizzed past but now the tracks seem to be taking you into a forest.

You smile as the trees have successfully broken up the monotony just a bit.

You remember that you brought a sleeping mask with you, along with earplugs.

It might be nice to get a short nap before you reach your destination.

You place your various sleep accouterment on your face, blocking out all other distractions.

The only sensation you feel is the steady movement of the train, which you find oddly comforting.

You awake to a poke.

Someone has let you know that it is time to exit the train.

You have never taken such a mode of transportation, so you intend to thank the kind stranger.

You were just a moment too late by the time you are able to remove your mask and catch your bearings.

The mystery helper has moved up the line, never to be found out.

You only brought a backpack with you, because you don't need very much for your day.

You happily make your way up to the front of the train and out into the station.

There is a bike rental stand, just like your friend said there would be.

You immediately make your way over to the bearded man running the stand, telling him that Jerry sent you.

The man is mischievous and pretends not to know Jerry before handing you a map and a lock.

Your bicycle is a sharp-looking royal blue beast.

One look at this machine and you know you are ready to take on your journey into nature.
Jerry had described the short journey as "transformative," and you were in desperate need of transformation.

As you find the road, you remember that you haven't ridden a bike in some time.

You do your best the mount the monstrosity but you're a little wobbly.

Soon the muscle memory of your childhood kicks back in and you are gliding down the street with the wind in your hair.

You find yourself riding through a sunny residential street.

There are children outside playing games while adults look on.

Birds are chirping as you pass along a road after road.

You are in search of something and you still have a long way to go.

There is a place within this city that only the locals know of.

It overlooks a breathtaking coastal region.

Finding this hidden gem is going to take some ingenuity on your part, but luckily your friend has given you very careful instructions to follow.

The city itself is lovely, and you'll enjoy your day regardless of your success.

You begin biking through side streets.

There are so many beautiful old buildings that have stood in their place for over a century.

The antiquated brick structures have been worn down by the hands of time but retain a measure of their former elegance.

The wind on this hot day is a welcome reprieve from the stagnant summer air.

You are passing so many smiling strangers, as the residential area slowly turns itself into the bustling city.

The various shops are becoming closer and closer together.

You are beginning to weave through people and cars as they navigate their way through the city.

Savory smells tempt you, as you pass street vendors.
The aroma reminds you briefly of childhood trips to the fair.

The point of your adventure was to find a place of silent beauty, but the roar of the city is just a different side of the same coin.

Watching others entwined in the mechanisms of their lives can also be fascinating.

You are allowed a brief snapshot of a stranger's day.

Their drama and their joy leak through the edges of these mental photographs.

So much information about these people is left up to interpretation.

Unfortunately, this is not a task that you have time to indulge in.

The street that your friend told you to find looks like any other.

There is nothing particularly special about this area.

You sit upon your bicycle gazing at a normal city block packed with buildings that are all squished together and connected.

Shops, apartments, and businesses share common walls.

You venture slowly down this street, in search of an apartment with a red door.

When you spot the building, it looks so unassuming that you almost consider turning back.

Suddenly it strikes you how crazy it's going to be to knock on a stranger's door and ask for access to their back yard.

You take a deep breath and gather your courage.

The door opens just before your close fist makes contact.

There is a rather small elderly lady with a barking dog behind her.

You are so nervous that you aren't able to speak, but luckily, she already knows exactly what you want.

The tiny old lady smirks and holds out an expectant hand.

You remember that your friend told you to pay her.

You shakily hand her a twenty and she opens her door for you.

The woman gives you a speech that you can tell she has made a thousand times in the past.
You are told that you are going to come across an old cement staircase with a guard railing on the side.

You are to jump over this and then squeeze between a wall and a stone.

Follow the path until you reach the top.

Don't follow the trail to the left.

You are sent on your way.

Her backyard is overgrown and unkempt.

You suspect that she keeps it in disrepair to hide the entrance to the old path.
You also have a sneaking suspicion that all of this is slightly less than legal.

This is a tourist city.

People flock from all over the world for a chance to see the strange coast.

The trail that you are walking now used to lead to the most scenic overlook in the area.

The city shut this attraction down long ago, and the path became overgrown and lost to the public.

Eventually, a house was built in front of this trail.

When the lady discovered that she had access to such a commodity, she began charging others to venture through her backyard.

Her business operated through word of mouth (and probably shady online advertisement).

You ignore the fact that it feels as though you have just completed a drug deal in secret as you progress along the path.

Trees with long strands of dangling ivy surround you.

The area has completely changed from city to jungle in a matter of steps.

You walk for what seems like an eternity, passing over the staircase.

The jump is slightly dangerous, but you handle the obstacle like a champion.

The squeezing portion of the journey is a bit scarier, but you remind yourself that the vista will be worth the trouble.

The wild forest and narrowing path make you nervous that perhaps you have lost your way.

Maybe this was all a giant set-up and you will be robbed now?

The trail has been twisting and turning as you trudge up an incline.

It seems as though you have been going up the side of a mountain.

At long last, you reach the overlook.

There is a concrete platform that is lined with a coal-colored wrought iron railing.

As you approach, your breath is taken away by the view of the coast.

Massive limestone structures jutting out from the emerald ocean waters.

These rocks shoot straight into the air.

They like pale skyscrapers ascending from the ocean floor.

The structures look like jagged stone titans watching over the shoreline.

The city was built to gawk at these natural marvels.

You sit and stare in awe.

You have never had such a perfect view of such beauty.

You are completely alone, at this moment.

You sit in quiet reflection, waiting for the sunset to bathe the stone giants in her heavenly neon glow.

Your trek has been worth every moment of fear or worry, and those emotions melt away from you now.

These stoic stone watchers remind of the absolute power that mother nature wields.

Rocks and cliffsides dwarf us in size.

We can only admire the vision behind such mysterious formations.

Absorbing ourselves in natural beauty can encourage a connection with our own mind by stripping away our trivial thoughts.

We are given to being caught up in the moment, in the majesty of our planet.

Chapter 23: The Spirit Source

That Wednesday made Quentin decide for sure: he needed to get away from the post office for a while.

As a mailman, Quentin got to spend quite a bit of time outside of the building already. On days like that, however, his ability to come and go only made his times inside the place even worse by comparison.

Nothing, in particular, could be pointed to that explained his decision to use a week of vacation days. The operations of the place were just the same as normal. He was returning a heavy package that the recipient hasn't shown up to receive. On that day, like many days, it kind of became his problem that they weren't present to take the package. Quentin gave the returns expert the package and asked her to mark it appropriately for the next upcoming delivery.

For the umpteenth time in a row, she could not figure out how to do this simple task. He couldn't help her fix this — it wasn't part of the training he had received, so he just didn't know how to. After going through this same monotony so many times, Quentin didn't think he would be able to go on much longer without quitting. He filled the required paperwork and told everyone he would see them the week after.

The job wasn't full of pain, toil, or even much discomfort. What he did have to deal with was repetitive errors and general boredom. He knew it wasn't the worst job by any stretch of the imagination, but he knew he couldn't work there the next day. He needed time away.

The last fifteen years had been a full experience if not all that exciting. He had now worked at the post office for half of his life; he had started as a desk attendant in high school, and now he was transporting packages to people every day at 30-years-old. Many would still consider him young, but after doing the same job for so long, he didn't feel particularly young.

In fact, sometimes he felt like he was an old man already, and that wasn't something he liked. He wanted to feel his age. It was hard to do when all you saw yourself doing for the rest of your life were the same repetitive tasks he had been doing for over a decade.

He didn't know what he was going to do during this vacation week, but one thing was for sure. He needed to give himself some quiet time alone so he could think about... anything.

Quentin didn't know what his goal was. He just knew that he wasn't going to work for a little while, and that time had to be spent figuring out exactly why he needed it.

Driving home after work felt a lot different when he knew he wouldn't be coming back for a long time. The possibilities were overwhelming when he thought about them. He had some extra money; he had a full week to do whatever he wanted. What would it be?

Without even trying, he found himself getting into habits despite the fact he told himself he wanted time to think. Quentin acted like he was going to worry the next day when he got home even though it wouldn't be for another seven days. When he automatically powered on his computer and played his online strategy game, he was cursing himself all the while.

Then again, it made sense that he wouldn't be able to break out of an old habit so easily. Every time Quentin got home, this is that he did. He didn't even do it on purpose anymore. It was muscle memory.

When he posted his first game, he groaned and shut down the computer. He wasn't groaning because he lost; he was groaning because he was disappointed with himself. Not only that, but he was mad at the "system" for creating an environment that led to habits like this.

Quentin didn't like the fact that his job had taken over his life so much that he did the same after-work activity when he literally had a full week to think more deeply about his life. He didn't even have to do it at home if he didn't want to. He could splurge on plane tickets and travel.

For a moment, he thought he would start now. He closed his eyes and had too many things to pay attention to. One of them stood out: why do I need so much noise all the time?

It was no surprise that his brain had a thought like this when he lived the way he did. Quentin practically drowned himself in noise on a constant and daily basis, but he had noticed this for some time now. He was a self-aware guy, no matter how many flaws he had.

He knew what was going on with him. Quentin was not oblivious, that was for certain. He could read social cues like a map, and when one of his major flaws got in the way of one of his goals, he was very much aware of it.

He surrounded himself with noise because he was an audiophile— he loved listening to music. It didn't feel right to him when there wasn't music for him to listen to, even in the background.

As he tried to think more deeply, he wondered if the real reason for his love for music was not as a true connoisseur, but as a guy who didn't want to think about his problems. While music was playing, he didn't have to hear himself think. He didn't have to hear his thoughts about the endlessness of work and his feeling of unfulfillment there. Quentin would rather have gone home every day and mask the thoughts with music rather than really deal with them. He knew it wasn't sustainable.

He had an idea. It was a small goal, but a novel one for him. He was going to prepare his food for dinner, but he wouldn't listen to any music while he did it. Quentin would just let whatever thoughts occurred to him occur to him as he did this.

The aroma of the frozen pizza coming out of the oven seemed much more potent when it wasn't being competed against by the blaring music on his headphones. He thought it tasted better, too. In just minutes, he scarfed it down and was back to square one. Here he was alone in the writer with his thoughts, enough money to do a lot of things, and an entire week to spend it. But he had no clue what he was going to do.

Quentin passed by fifteen minutes by staring at his shoes at the front door of the house. He saw a lot of things about it that had never occurred to him before. For one thing, the shoelaces seemed awfully long — a lot longer than he saw them to be when he wore them every day. Also, their orange color was a lot darker than he thought it was.

He hadn't drunk coffee or done anything of the kind; he thought it had to be the sound deprivation that was making him see the world differently. Even without paying attention to his surroundings, he was noticing things happening that were different from before. He had a clearer head than he had had in a long time. He couldn't believe it was just from taking off his headphones.

Then the second thought stood out to him since he took off his headphones: **I need a purpose.**

The thought surprised him and didn't surprise him at the same time. It surprised him because of the medium through which he heard yet another clear thought; he usually saw his mind as something that was under his control, but when he heard these thoughts, it didn't feel like he had them actively. He almost felt like a passive observer of his own thoughts. It didn't startle him per se, but he certainly took note of the sharing.

The question didn't surprise him because he thought about that question all the time while he was working. When he drove from house to house, delivering mail and trying to deliver packages, he often wondered if this work would be his legacy on this planet.

Like all things in his life, he didn't see it as a completely bad thing, but he did feel an unmistakable feeling of dissatisfaction from the things he did every day. He could rationally expect to make good enough money to retire comfortably if he kept working here. But then he would never become anything else. He would stay at the same level of intelligence, courage, maturity. He had a thought for how to sum up his feelings on the matter: this was enough, but maybe enough was not enough.

He felt his body moving towards the coat rack. It reminded him of when he had thoughts that felt like they happened to him instead of ones he felt like he was creating: he didn't will himself to get his jacket, he simply found himself doing it. Apparently, he was leaving the house.

When he stepped outside the house, the rain fell much more lightly than on his way home. If he was honest with himself, he hasn't even thought about the rain on his way here, because he was so distracted by the tunes playing in his ears.

Being outside in the rain seemed a lot different when he wasn't playing music. For one thing, it was louder than he remembered. He stepped instead a small puddle and was surprised at how distinctive the sound of the splash was.

His body may have propelled him to come out here, but once he was in his car, driving through the neighborhood, it was clear that he had no plan for what to do next. He was going to have to come up with something on his own.

Since he already ate, he didn't feel like getting food. But he lived in a pretty rural place, so there wasn't much he could do out here. After a little bit of thinking, he thought maybe he could follow suit with not having music on and do an activity with low sensory stimulation. There was a park down the road from the entrance to the neighborhood; he could go there and look at the stars.

Going to the park alone at night felt strange, but it was something for him to do, somewhere to go. Today probably had to be strange, he thought. He had been questioning more and more lately, whether sticking with his safe, comfortable job was the thing he should do. He would have to spend some more time with himself if he was going to find answers.

As he took a seat at the table in the park, he became strongly aware of how important it was that things stayed quiet right now. He had barely processed his thought to turn off the music through the music he had been playing basically non-stop for years. From there, he realized that he needed to find a purpose. His present lifestyle and livelihood were not enough to fulfill his deeper needs.

He had a lot going through his head now that it was quiet, but one thought seemed most salient, and it was telling him that he shouldn't be listening to music that constantly anymore. Quentin couldn't go against that, because listening to his own thoughts had gotten him this far.

He didn't know a lot about the stars, but an ex had taught him some of the basic constellations. Out here in the country, he was able to see a lot more of them than people who lived in the city. He tried to find the Big Dipper as his minds processed this.

There was a new thing that began to occupy his mind as he looked at the stars. He didn't want today to be an exception to a long-established way of living. He wanted to keep up his peace from the noise that used to play in his ears at all times. There was a way he could think of to take care of that, but he didn't want to do it.

For a long time, he didn't do anything or pursue the line of thinking any further. He simply enjoyed his time sitting on top of the table at the park. When no other strategy came to mind, he knew this was what he had to do.

He knew there was no alternative way that he could make sure this difference he was feeling would last. If he didn't do it, tomorrow everything would go back to the way things were before. With some regret but no hesitation, Quentin walked back to his car and went home. What he was about to do wasn't easy, but it was necessary.

At first, his plan was to throw it all away. But there were some problems with this. For one, doing that would be wasteful. The materials would be harmful to the environment.

But also, even though it sometimes felt like he made quite a lot since he was only supporting himself, he didn't want to kid himself about how much money he had. He ultimately decided to sell the electronics in his house instead of tossing them out.

He would have to do it in the morning, though, because at the moment everything was closed. He had a nightly routine of listening to soothing music to get to bed, but he wouldn't be able to do it that night without throwing off all the changes he was trying to make, so he didn't play anything that night.

It felt like he didn't need to, anyway. There was this feeling that he had had a productive day, and that feeling made it quite easy to fall asleep. Not only that, but he knew there was a lot to look forward to over this next week, which gave him a sense of calm. When Quentin closed his eyes, it didn't take long for him to start dreaming.

In his dream, he was hovering in the sky at night when the stars were out. The stars kept switching positions, and he watched them play their celestial game of musical chairs. It felt good to be next to their radiant energy.

But then he started to be overwhelmed by it. Slowly, the light overtook his vision, and soon enough, he wasn't able to see anything. That was when he woke up.

When he was awake, he didn't mind it so much, though. It wasn't exactly a bad dream; he had just lost his vision, and then he woke up. He slowly regained his vision now as his eyes started to open up.

Then, he started on the task he had given himself for that day. There was no rush for him to do it, because there were still six more days after today. Even if he wanted to get on a plane somewhere, he still had time to do it. He didn't stress himself out over this; the whole reason he had taken a vacation was so he could get away from stress like that.

The truth was, Quentin didn't know that much about any of the gadgets he had. They were just things he bought and liked to use. He didn't know how to fix something whose battery stopped charging. When he dropped something, he couldn't repair it by himself. He had no choice but to pay someone to fix it or buy a new one.

For this reason, he didn't feel exactly comfortable going into the store to sell all his stuff. People tended to look at him and assume he knew a lot of gadgets, and he just didn't.

Of course, he couldn't sell everything. He still needed his phone, so he could keep in contact with his friends and family. He thought it was still a good idea to keep a laptop. But besides that, most everything else could go.

He was a little unsure about selling his television, but he felt like he had to be consistent if he was going to do this at all. So in multiple trips, he brought his TV, gaming systems, headphones, desktop computer, and all the miscellaneous wires.

When he was all done, Quentin felt strangely relieved. He was expecting this all to be a lot more painful for him, but it wasn't. He knew he had done something that was good for him in the long run, and it gave him a satisfaction that he hadn't gotten in a good while.

It was funny how much easier it was to go home without all those electronics slowing him down. Carrying things into his car one trip at a time and then into the store one at a time was as tedious as his job. But when he got home, he didn't have anything but his laptop and phone at home.

Despite being accustomed to spending a lot of time on his gadgets, Quentin didn't think he was at risk for starting to spend a lot of time on his phone or laptop now.

Those two were never things that he wasted time on; he never took any interest in downloading apps on his phone, and there wasn't a lot he could do on his old laptop. He still had a shelf full of books he had never read, so he felt like he still had a lot he could do.

He even felt cleaner without all of those devices, creating heat and making him sweat. The dust that used to get on them wasn't in the air anymore. There was now empty space where his stuff used to be.

Before getting into a book, he stared at the naked spot on the floor where his entertainment center used to be. He had thrown it out after selling the TV because he wouldn't have a use for it anymore; it was just taking up space. He liked the way it looked with nothing on it.

When he started reading his book, he made an observation that reading was a lot like looking at an empty space. He read a story about a knight who fell a monster, and all of it seemed real to him. But in reality, it all came together through words alone.

Quentin wanted to see himself in the knight, but the story didn't give him anything he could cling onto to justify that. Compared to this hero with a dragon-slaying sword, he felt like he hadn't done anything with his life. He hadn't slain any creatures; he barely even knew how to handle it when a bat got into his house.

Then he finished reading the story, and all it left him with were thoughts like this. He may have been able to take the place of the knight while he was reading the story, but now that it was over, they didn't have enough in common for him to do that.

He had to grapple with the fact that reading was one more way he used to distract himself when he still hadn't decided what his purpose was. He hadn't decided if he would go back to his job as a mailman or not. His brain told him it was the smart thing to do, but Quentin didn't think the "smart" thing made him happy.

As far as he could tell, though, there was nothing he could replace this boring job with. He had no idea how he would figure it out. He thought the answer might have come to him from getting into a good book, but all the knight's tale had done was fill him with feelings of inadequacy.

No one ever taught him how to deal with this problem. All anyone ever talked about were things happening right now. They didn't look into the future and what might happen then, and when he thought about it, that was the thing that bothered him. Looking into the future was what caused him to take a week off in the first place. It wasn't really that he couldn't have gone in to work the next day, because he could have.

The problem was, he didn't think he would be able to go to work tomorrow a year from today. And the year after that.

When he reflected on it, he should have thought about the future more, instead of waiting until he was in his thirties. But he had been so mesmerized by the music playing in his headphones that he never gave himself the mental space to think.

But even with most of his gadgets gone, he didn't see any real direction for finding the answer he was looking for. He thought everything would be clear to him once they were sold. While his thoughts did feel less cluttered without them here, there seemed to still be a fundamental problem.

It was this house. So long as he stayed in here, no matter what things he had in it, he couldn't think clearly and find the meaning he had been searching for. This house was the place where he had let all his bad habits continue. Staying here would not make real change possible.

But what was he supposed to do? Quentin didn't have any other leads for careers. People couldn't just drop their whole lives for something new just like that, and there was a reason for it. If he wasn't doing anything else with his life but delivering mail and wasting time at home, it had to be because he wasn't able to do anything else.

Just like that, he felt his body move on its own for the second time since yesterday. He was once again propelled to various places around his house. He threw all his important things in a backpack like clothes, paperwork, and money. Then, he felt himself walking outside and into his car.

His hand turned the ignition, and his foot turned on the gas. He steered out of his driveway and drove in the direction of the interstate.

Even when he felt as out of control as he did now, Quentin didn't feel any stress. He knew what he was doing, although he didn't understand it. He was driving towards the highway, and around here, the only place that went was the airport. Apparently, he was going to fly somewhere. He just didn't know where yet.

After paying for parking and finding his way inside, he had to decide what came next. He thought for a moment that it wouldn't be possible to fly internationally, because he didn't have a passport. But on second thought, he did have a passport card, so there were two places he could go: Canada and Mexico. He wasn't sure his body could handle the extreme change of temperature from there to Mexico, so Canada it was.

He wondered if he should have visited his family instead, but he realized that wasn't going to help him find his purpose. Quentin was on his own journey. Being around people who already had expectations of who he was wouldn't help him discover who he really was — it would only make him more and more like the guy everyone already saw him as. Looking at his available options for his chosen country, he decided to fly to Montreal.

Quentin had never flown a plane before. He was shocked at what a slow process it was just to get to the gate. He also thought the plane would take off soon after he sat down, and that didn't turn out to be the case at all. Soon enough, though, the plane took off, and his adventure could begin.

He felt amazed at how his body had taken him here. It wasn't as if he had planned for this to happen. He didn't make a plan this morning to get on a plane, but now here he was, soaring through the sky like it was nothing.

The other people in the plane didn't seem to recognize the magic of it. They were busy watching the in-flight movie and looking at their devices.

Quentin stared out the window for nearly the entire trip. Seeing the wing outside did make him a little queasy — it was a reminder that they were in the air, and also that he wouldn't be able to leave until they landed. But his pure joy about being in the sky overrode any anxiety he may have felt. This journey was only going to be about an hour, anyway, so he didn't have to wait long.

How could it be that he felt out of control of ending up here, yet he felt totally in control of his thoughts reacting to it? It was a mystery to him, and he didn't think he was ever going to solve it.

When they finally landed, Quentin scuttled out of the airport like everyone else. He used the airport taxi service to have someone drive him into the city. He didn't have any plans for lodging; it was something he was going to have to figure out eventually, but the sky wasn't even dark yet. He would think about it when the time was right.

Quentin didn't know anything about Montreal prior to this trip. Seeing French at the top of every sign, along with English, was not something he expected to see. He didn't have any expectations.

While he was tempted many times to use his phone to find a tourist attraction, he didn't want to revert back to old patterns. Quentin decided to simply walk around and find a place in real life instead of on the screen.

Since he was at a loss of what to do first, he went into a champagne bar and ordered a glass. He didn't drink but a few times a year if that, but he did like a nice drink every once in a blue moon. When he was finished with it, he went back out into the street and tried to follow the lead of other people who looked like tourists.

When Quentin did this, he eventually happened upon the Montreal Museum of Fine Arts. He came from a family of artists, and he was really the only one who didn't partake in any of them, but coming from such a family did teach him an admiration for painting, sculpture, and drawing.

In most situations, he wouldn't have liked a place like this museum. The people here came off as a bit stuffy. They were wearing much nicer clothes than he was. Today he didn't seem to mind, though. He actually liked how quiet everyone was in here. It made him think of the peace he felt at home when he took off the headphones and sold the devices, but he didn't feel trapped in his old habits here like he did at home.

He spent most of his time there in one room in particular. The walls were painted to look like they were in a forest. The framed paintings on the walls were supposed to be the draw, but Quentin found himself looking at the trees instead.

Then he sighed, remembering he was supposed to be finding his purpose here. Maybe he was losing himself in these painted trees in the same way he lost himself in his music and gadgets. Maybe it wasn't any different.

The next place everywhere was walking towards was the Notre Dame replica, the Notre Dame Basilica. This was a place Quentin could have more personal attachment to because history had always been his favorite subject.

People were even quieter in this cathedral, although they didn't need to be. The inside was so vast that no one would be able to hear them. Whether people were speaking in English or French, they did so quietly. Quentin wished he had someone to enjoy this trip with, but he reminded himself yet again that he was on his own journey.

Just as he had lost himself in the painted trees at the art museum, he recognized that he forgot himself in admiring the architecture of this place.

But he finally stopped himself. What was so bad about making something so beautiful overtake his conscious experience? Perhaps letting go of his conscious thought for pure sensory enjoyment was not such a bad thing.

No matter what he did, Quentin was going to go between thinking about himself and forgetting himself for the images that came into his senses. He thought that maybe he didn't need a "purpose" as long as he had this understanding. He could continue to grow as a man and keep finding new things to love. But rushing himself to reach a goal when he didn't know what that meant would only make him unhappy.

Quentin wasn't sure how long it was going to last, but he thought he would stay in Montreal a bit longer than a week. Sure, he would lose his job back home, but going back to it didn't feel like a real option anyway. Going back would just bring him back through the whole cycle again.

All he was concerned about was today. And today, he was going to seek out a friend. Quentin had friends back home, but no one to whom he could show his full self. Now that he was in a new place where people didn't know him, he could reinvent himself. He didn't know who that would be — himself or the friend. Hopefully, he would find someone who would let him sleep on their couch a little while until he found some footing here.

Chapter 24: A Mysterious Place

A cave is always such a mysterious place.

A cave is where you will find buried treasures and unlikely beauty.

A cave can also be the place deep inside of you where you hide all of your deepest desires and darkest fears.

In your next bedtime story and guided meditation, you will travel to a hidden cave of mystery to find just what your mind, heart, and soul need in order for you to feel free, relaxed, and relieved.

Begin by finding your most comfortable position.

If you are preparing for bed and ready for this bedtime story, make sure you have everything you will need to feel settled.

As you get comfortable in your space, connect to your breath and begin to listen to the flow of air being pulled in through your nostrils, being held in your chest for a moment's pause, and releasing your breath in one, long exhale.

Breathe in again, pulling in clarity, calmness, serenity, hold it here in your lungs, and exhale it out.

Breathe like this for a few moments and make any final adjustments you need to to find the most comfortable position for your body.

As you breathe in and out, connect to your sense and feeling.

How is your body feeling right now?

Where do you feel stiffness, soreness, achiness?

Where do you feel tightness, or like you are holding onto something that needs to be released?

When you find these spaces in your body, breathe into them with your inhale, filling the space with clean, clear oxygen.

Hold the breath in this area for a moment, and release it slowly and steadily out.

Again, find these spaces of tension, of soreness, or tightness.

Breathe long, slow, soothing breaths into these areas, hold the breath here for a moment and then let it all out in a long, steady exhale.

Feel your body becoming heavier and more relaxed as you breathe out your tension.

Feel your body sinking more deeply into the relaxed position you are lying in right now.

Feel your body acclimate to this restful state.

Notice how it feels when it is free of tension.

Notice how it feels after focused breathing.

Your body and mind are linked. It is one.

Everything that you think, your body can hear it, feel it, sense it.

All of your emotions, your dears, your anxieties, all of your trauma, sadness, frustration, all of these things become a part of your physical self.

All of these mental patterns and beliefs become a part of your physical form, the way you carry yourself, the way your shoulders and neck tighten.

Continue to breathe in and out and feel your body melt and become relaxed, like honey dripping from a honeycomb.

See your muscles and ligaments, joints, and bones, becoming thick and fluid-like golden honey.

Feel your body relaxing in this way with every release of tension or tightness as you exhale slowly.

Now, once upon a time, you saw a starry night.

It was the first thing you saw when you opened your inner eye.

In your mind, see the starry night sky.

You are there now.

You are laying underneath a great, wide expanse of stars.

The sky is rich and full of these burning bulbs, millions of miles away.

You are in a place where you can see all of the stars of the night sky.

It is the only light.

Your body is calm and liquid, and your mind is seeing this space, this expanse of stars.

Your energy can feel the power of this starlight beaming down and touching the landscape that surrounds you, wherever you are lying.

This starry sky reaches across and over everything, as far as your eye can see, from horizon to horizon.

There is no end to it.

What kind of landscape do you find yourself in?

A desert canyon?

A pine forest?

A meadow?

A prairie?

Where did your mind transport you to view this starry night sky?

Look around inside your mind at this space.

What lies beneath the sky of stars, other than your body?

It can be anything and everything you can imagine…

This place you are in, it is real.

It exists inside of you.

It is a place that your mind can see and that you can travel to with your consciousness.

You can see it change and evolve as you change and evolve, and it will always contain everything you need to explore your deeper mind.

This is your conscious reality in your unconscious mind space.

Take it in and let it be whatever comes to your mind.

This space you are in has always existed and always will.

It is a place of good intentions and dreams.

It is a place of fearlessness and awakening.

It is a place you will go to whenever you need to find what you are looking for to help you forward on your healing path.

Let it begin to take new shape in your mind as it changes from starry night to dawn's light.

See the sun rising on a horizon, bringing new energy to this landscape.

As the sun begins to rise, you can begin to walk toward the pink and orange light of sunrise.

Let your body float across the landscape, continuing to feel fluid like honey.

Feel yourself being naturally guided and carried forward in this landscape of your inner mind and thoughts.

Let the world around you take new shape as you gently explore its features.

You are walking to a distant space near the horizon.

You see far off in the distance a flickering light.

You are drawn to it like a bee to pollen, or a moth to a flame.

You walk toward it.

As you get closer and closer, the dawn turns into day, and the day turns to dusk, and the dusk turns to night again, blanketing the night sky with stars as far as the eye can see.

The flickering light is now close to you.

As you draw nearer under the stars, you see that it is a campfire that someone built and left all alone.

As you come closer to it, you feel its warmth and the orange glow on your cheeks.

It feels good to be here under the stars in this land next to the warm, passionate glow of the fire.

You can hear the crack and hiss of the burning embers, and you feel this fire awakening within you, warming you from your very core, aligning with your own burning flame.

This fire you found under the stars is a reflection of your internal flame.

How does your internal flame feel today?

Is it burning brightly?

Does it lack fuel?

Do you feel it growing as you relax in this inner landscape?

Take a deep breath in and allow the power of flame to fill your soul, warming the liquid honey of your body.

Exhale slowly and look out into the distance, all-around your inner world, feeling the calm of everything you have created in your subconscious wilderness.

Underneath this starry night, the world is full of hidden mysteries and secrets to be unearthed.

Your greatest desires and needs are here in this place.

Can you look for them here?

Can you sense which direction you need to walk to find your hidden cave of answers?

Let yourself feel pulled forward in a direction.

Walk away from the glow of the firelight and let yourself journey toward this hidden place that is waiting for you to come to it, to show up.

Continue your journey, breathing softly and deeply, letting the radiance of each star glimmer on your skin from far off in the galaxy.

Let your honey-body glide and float without any tension or fear.

See the place where you know the cave might be hidden and follow your path there.

Your path to this cave can be anything you want.

As you draw nearer to where you feel pulled, you find yourself in a canyon with high rock walls.

Let your mind fill in this space with color, with detail, with scope.

This rocky canyon holds many deep mysteries and energies from deep within your mind.

As you walk through this canyon, you are still being pulled toward this source of power, somewhere hidden, deep in the caves of your consciousness.

It's somewhere here, the opening.

It blends in so well to the rock walls because you are so good at keeping it safe and hidden from others.

You are looking for the opening of the cave when you spot a small stone on the surface where you are gliding.

The stone is a beautiful color and is perfectly smooth.

It fits in your palm and feels like a comfortable and soothing weight.

Its cool exterior warms in the palm of your hand.

You notice its color and its shape as you hold it, and somehow you know that this stone is the key to finding the hidden cave.

This stone marks the entrance somewhere close by.

In your eye, you can see the possibilities of where this hidden entrance might be.

You can glance around now and try to spot it.

Look for a sign that will show you the path to the hidden entrance.

Is it another colorful stone marking the gateway?

Is it perhaps a secret message carved in the rock wall?

Seek the sign to show you the door to the cave.

Welcome the energy of the cave by finding the entrance.

The entrance will become obvious once you see it, and once you see it, it opens wide for you, like the mouth of a yawning lion.

You can see the tunnel that opens into the deep of this canyon wall.

You are free to walk toward it and enter the mysteries that are hidden here.

Are you ready to walk the path?

There is nothing to fear as you enter the tunnel of the cave.

It is open and welcoming to you. It is a part of your thoughts, your soul, your mind.

It feels right.

It feels natural.

It is a place within you that is hiding something of great value to you on your journey of healing and self-discovery.

Let yourself flow into the tunnel opening of the cave and follow the path.

You can see where you are going because the walls of the cave are glittering and alive with bioluminescence.

Blue-green light, purple light, white light, shimmers from the life forms that grow in this magic place.

You are being shown the way down your path by this organic light source, and you are brave enough to keep walking straight through the winding and crooked pathways carved into the walls of the cave.

There is nowhere inside where you will be stuck or won't be able to get out.

This cave is a friend to you and your sense of self.

It is a part of you, this cave.

It is a reflection of your subconscious thoughts and feelings.

Let it become what it wants to be so that you can see your true mind inside of the shadows of this cave.

You are nearing an opening, a large chamber at the center of the cave maze.

You can feel the air opening up here.

You can hear the echo of dripping water hitting the floor of the cave as it falls from stalactites growing off the ceiling, hanging down like chandeliers of water and light.

There are crystals growing in all directions in this chamber, adding to the light of the space.

They are white, clear, purple, and other colors of quartz growing out of walls, the cave floor, the ceiling.

You are surrounded by the vibration of these crystals.

You can feel them humming in soft tones, filling the space with the frequency of love.

You are safe and guarded by the energy of this space.

As you walk into the center of the cave, surrounded by all of the crystals, you see a large wooden chest with a lock on it.

The lock is in the shape of the colorful stone you found outside the cave opening.

You can open this wooden chest with the colorful rock that showed you where to find the hidden cave.

You approach the wooden chest and kneel on the floor in front of it.

Notice its features.

How big is it?

How worn and used?

What does it fell like when you touch it?

Take a deep breath in and consider what this chest feels like to you on the outside, exhaling as you reflect on it.

Inhale again and consider what might be locked inside.

What is within this chest hidden in your cave of mysterious?

What have you come to find?

What are you looking for that you didn't even realize was hidden?

Take a moment to reflect in this space, surrounded by crystals and bioluminescence.

Breathe gently and slowly, in and out.

Consider what you need to open in your life, something buried deep within that needs to come to the surface that needs to be awakened in your everyday existence.

You have a colorful stone with you.

It is in the palm of your hand.

You can open the lock of the chest with the stone.

The stone slides snugly into an opening in this strange lock.

You hear it click open and fall from the chest onto the cave floor.

The chest is now unlocked, and you can look inside to find what you need right now.

All you have to do is lift the lid and look inside.

Let it come to you naturally.

Do not guess.

Let the hidden item, or emotion, or memory, or experience, organically take shape as you open the chest and look inside.

If it takes a moment to materialize, that's okay.

It might be a small object.

It could be an entire person, you know.

It might look like a symbol of what you want or desire.

Only you will know.

Only you can see it.

Take a few moments to look inside the chest and find the hidden gift.

Whatever it is, it is now time for you to look at it in the cave.

If you find something you were not expecting, you are on the right track.

If you found something you were expecting to find, then you are also on the right track.

The hidden cave of mysterious shows you what you need to see right now, today, to help you align with your higher purpose, your wholeness, your growth.

Whatever you have found in this treasure chest is what will help you heal and find peacefulness from within.

It could be a lost passion or a hidden desire.

It could be a relationship that needs to end or begin anew.

It could be a profession that has been calling to you for years or a career that is at a dead end.

It could be an old object from childhood that is the key to rekindling your childlike curiosity.

It could be a memory that hides your greatest pain or your deepest love.

It is time to acknowledge your feelings about this hidden truth.

It is time to accept what it is you are hiding or blocking from being seen or heard, or recognized.

This hidden artifact of your subconscious mind is asking to be held by you, is asking to be given more attention.

Whatever emotions are connected to it, any beliefs or attitudes that might come up with it, are important to see also.

Let yourself spend time examining this hidden energy that you have kept locked in this hidden cave deep within your mind.

This energy that you have held onto is ready to be shown out of the cave, to be bathed in the starlight and the rising dawn.

You can shrink it down and hold it in your hand, carrying the essence of it out of the cave with you.

You can close the lid of the trunk and lock it again.

You will return to it again sometime soon, and it will contain another hidden treasure for you to open.

Let your breath relax you as you begin your ascent out of the cave, touching the giant crystals to give you balance along the way, soaking in the subtle glow of the bioluminescent organisms clinging to the cave walls, lighting your way out.

The cave is narrowing behind you as you exit, hiding again until it is time for your return.

The opening of the cave closes as you take your final step back out into the canyon, like the jaws of the yawning lion closing again.

You are back underneath the starlight, and you are holding the essence of your hidden mystery in your hand.

In your other hand, the colorful stone is warm and weighted.

You drop it on the ground and leave it there for your next visit, carrying only the essence of your hidden mystery in your hand.

It is time to let it see the light of day, out of the cave walls, out of the buried and locked chest.

Hold this energy in your hand and carry it with you through the canyon, following the starlight as it changes into a morning sunrise.

You can see the flickering campfire still flickering with life on the distant horizon.

Walk to it, breathing in gently and softly, relaxing your body, keeping it like honey flowing smoothly.

As you near the fire, you approach it with good intentions.

This hidden secret you have locked inside of you is ready to be transformed.

It is time to give it to the light and let it evolve and grow in the way it asks to, as you welcome it into your higher consciousness.

Whatever you have pulled from the secret chest in the hidden cave, whether it is positive or negative, is asking to be turned over to the fire of the dawn.

Lifting your hand high, hold the essence of your hidden secret above the flames.

Hold it up to the disappearing starlight and the waking sun.

Show this energy that you found locked deep inside of you that you are ready to set it afire so that it can change so that it can grow so that it can go through metamorphosis.

You are ready to let your inner light shine brighter by giving this locked secret to the fire.

Take a deep breath in, slowly inhaling, filling yourself with empowered energy.

As you exhale, see yourself dropping the image or essence of your hidden mystery into the flames.

Hear it crackle and hiss.

Hear it burn and transform.

This is where you start fresh.

This is where you can begin anew.

You are ready to seek out new ideas, new energy, new comfort, just by letting go of this secret energy to the flame of creation, passion, and desire.

You are burning an opening into your journey so that you can have new momentum, new life-force, new excitement.

You can now relax as the sun comes forward and warms you like the flame you sit beside.

Lie down next to the fire.

Feel the starlight on your back and the dawn's light on your face.

Breathe in slowly and smoothly and give yourself the peace to relax and dream of what tomorrow will bring.

Feel the relief of knowing where to find your hidden cave anytime you need to resolve a buried intention.

Let yourself burrow into the earth where you are lying in front of the fire.

Relax.

Dream.

Rest.

Sleep.....

Breathing in Nature

Breath control can be useful in a variety of situations.

The practice allows your mind to calm itself when you are feeling overstimulated.

It can be a valuable precursor to meditation, allowing the thoughts from your day to fall away so that you are essentially a "clean slate."

The next time you find yourself enjoying the natural world, trying a breathing exercise.

It can add so much to your experience by allowing you to fully engage with your surroundings.

The following steps will allow you to embrace the stillness of the moment.

1. Sit, stand or lay in a comfortable position with your diaphragm unobstructed.
2. Bring your awareness to every individual muscle group in your body, starting with your feet. Feel your limbs and then relax them. Feel and then relax.
3. Pay attention to your breath as you inhale and then exhale. Feel the sensations in your chest or stomach, watch as your diaphragm expands and contracts.
4. Place one hand on your stomach and one on your chest. As you continue to breathe, allow yourself to deeply experience the changes in your diaphragm.
5. If you find yourself becoming distracted by errant thoughts, just refocus on the sound of your breath. You may also use a count of four on your inhale and exhale if that would better aid in concentration.

You can use this method for any reason, including building your focus.

The next time you find yourself sitting beneath a shady tree or enjoying a moment outside, try controlled breathing.

Remember to be kind to yourself with your thoughts drift unintentionally and appreciative toward yourself whenever you complete an exercise.

Chapter 25: Curiosity and the Cat

The man walked into the house, disturbing my sleep for the third time today. I supposed I could forgive him, as he looked nearly as unhappy about it as I did. What I wouldn't forgive, I decided, was how long it had been since my bowl was last filled. The water bowl was decently filled, but the food was lacking. As the man paced through the living room, I decided I would lodge a complaint and see if there was anything to be done about it.

I walked over to where he now sat in the foyer. He was doing something odd with his head. It looked like he was holding onto it so it wouldn't fall off his shoulders, but I didn't think they were prone to such mishaps. I knew my head wouldn't fall off of its own accord, but humans are different in many ways, as I had come to discover after living with them for many years.

I stepped over his feet as he sat, holding onto his head and rubbed up against his legs. Nasty smells on the man these days. We would have to rub for a while in order to neutralize that smell, but I knew he would just go right back out and wallow in whatever it was that made him smell that way. I cringed a little when he pet me, as the smell was all over him. Still, the contact felt nice and the heat of his hands was lovely.

"Now will you feed me?" I asked him. He mimicked the sound I made but made no moves to remedy the urgent situation in my bowl. I asked him once more, but I did so as I moved toward the kitchen this time.

"Oh, you need to be fed, don't you?" The man stood up from his perch. That was the ticket; he understood what was needed now.

I sat patiently by my bowl waiting for him to fill it. He milled about the kitchen, grabbing things of little consequence to me from various places. He seemed to be gathering some food of his own before putting mine together. I didn't know how long it had been since he had eaten, but I didn't really think I would know what to do with the information if I did know.

Eventually, the man filled my bowl and set about the task of eating the food he had prepared for himself as well. After I had finished eating, I thought I would search the house for the woman once again. She had been missing for what seemed like several days. Granted, I think I have a different sense of time than the humans in my house seem to have. They seemed to sleep so rarely, and they seemed to leave me for days at a time. Though, they were there at every feeding. They were there to feed me when it was light, and they were there to feed me when it was dark. Did it get dark on odd days and light on even? It tired me to think of such things.

In spite of my rather thorough search of the home, there were no signs that the woman had returned while I slept. Where had she gone? This was not ideal, having the woman leave the home. She was warm and she scratched that place I like behind my ears. The man scratched places too, but he was more of a petter than a scratcher.

Oh well, **I thought.** Perhaps the woman will return after my next sleep.

I awoke to a very strange noise sometime later. Something that sounded like the humans coming home, but there was something else with them. Another cat? No, it sounded wrong.

I sat by the door and waited for it to open. When it did, the man was holding a large basket of some kind and the woman was close behind.

"You've found her! Well done, human! Woman, you may scratch behind my ears as soon as you please. I thought you had gotten lost someplace when you weren't—" I had been interrupted by that strange-sounding basket the man had brought home. **How rude,** I thought to myself as I watched the man lower it to the ground.

The woman, who had lost weight since I had last seen her, hung her jacket up on the hook by the door. The man, who looked exhausted, hugged the woman. I stretched up onto my hind legs to peer into the basket. What had been making that racket I had heard coming from the front steps?

As I peered into the basket, I saw a moving... Well, I was fairly perplexed as to what it was at first. Its face was wrinkly, and it looked sad as it cooed. No, not sad. Sleepy? It quivered as it opened its mouth, wrinkled its face further, and sucked in. **Oh, it's yawning,** I thought. I looked at the humans, who were watching my investigation of their basket.

"Kiki, that's Elena; she's our baby. Isn't she precious?" I looked at the basket again, finally understanding what I was looking at. This was one of their young. Where were the rest of them? Had the woman lost the rest of her litter? I peered at the basket, wondering if I had perhaps overlooked one or more other young in the basket. No, it was just the one. I would have to read carefully around the woman for a while if only one of her litter was saved.

I left the kitten (what did humans call their young?) in its basket and addressed the humans directly.

"I wish you had told me to expect young in the home. I would have provided made provisions and hunted for you." I could tell by the look on the humans' faces that they understood. They always seemed to understand me when I spoke to them.

The man went into the kitchen to fill my bowl, then picked me up to carry me around for a moment. This was always slightly unsettling, but I enjoyed the closeness with the man.

The woman did the same with her young. I looked at the woman, sorry that she had gone through the troubles of labor without me there to care for her and give her warmth. I was proud of her, though, for bringing home the little survivor. There was hope for my humans yet, I thought.

Chapter 26: A Fantasy World

The afternoon sun shone brightly on the green leaves and green trees in the forests, it was like there was a big smile on its face. The birds chirped happily while the antelopes grazed lazily in the afternoon sun, and even the lions were all sitting peacefully, too lazy and full to hunt. On the land, everything was at peace. Things were quite different deep in the ocean and seas all over! The King of all the Mermaids and Mermen in seas and ocean all around was angry. His staff of authority had been stolen! The king's anger made the oceans hot, and if something was not done about it soon, the lives of all the sea and ocean creatures were in danger!

The day before, things had been really different. There had been a festival at the sea palace, and all Mermaids and Mermen had come from far and wide to celebrate the festival. It was an occasion that brought all Mermaids and Mermen together each year. They would all eat and drink at each other's houses. That is why a lot of Merfolk knew one another, in fact, even the Merfolk in the Oceans and the seas knew one another, they were all one big family.

The king was unmarried, so, on the festival days, Mermaids from all Oceans and Seas would dress as beautifully as possible. Maybe they would be lucky to have the king choose them.

All the other festivals had gone the same way, the king did not find any lady whom he liked. But this year's festival was different, the king had finally chosen a Mermaid to become his wife, and she was indeed beautiful!

In the morning of the festival, a Mermaid hurried from the Mermarket after buying all the supplies she would need to cook food for all the guests she would have that day. She opened the door to see her daughter fast asleep in the most unladylike manner. Her hands were piled up above her head, she had drool running from the left corner of her mouth, and her tail was unceremoniously falling off the couch. She patted her on her arm and said, "Geraldine honey, aren't you going to the festival? Leslie will soon be here you know".

Geraldine opened one of her baby blue eyes and swept her brunette hair out of her eyes while muttering, "C'mon mom, I need some me time, a girl needs her beauty sleep you know". Her mom chuckled as she watched her daughter roll off the couch and fall to the floor with a dull thud, then she swam off to wear her festival gown. Geraldine hurriedly rubbed some powder on her smooth face, ran her fingers through her hair and then used some cream to make her tail shiny. Then, she leapt off the chair to leave the house.

Geraldine rolled her eyes as her mom burst into laughter when she saw her appearance. Then, she dragged her back into the room, where she helped her to brush and pack her hair beautifully. After just a few minutes, Geraldine had become restless and wanted to leave. She never saw herself getting picked by the king anyway, so she did not understand why her mom always dressed her up so nicely each time. The last two festivals, Geraldine had slept off at old Merman Titus' house after she had eaten and she did not even visit the palace, much less see the king.

Her friend Leslie's knock saved her. She jumped off the chair and hurried off while yelling, "Bye mom". Then, she ran to meet her friend, and they left for the festival together. Geraldine hoped to see old Merman Titus so that she could eat another one of his sweet delicacies, but she was disappointed when they got to his house and found the door locked. She sighed and said to her friend, "Oh well, I guess I don't have a choice but to attend the festival, even though I know I'll be bored to death".

Leslie laughed, and they went on their way to the palace. They talked as they went on their way and a lot of Merfolk greeted Geraldine. She was quite popular, everyone knew her to be kind-hearted and very polite, although she was quite restless, she loved everyone around her. Whenever they needed help with their house chores, the older Merfolk always called Geraldine, and she would help them.

By the time they got to the palace, other girls had joined them including Tetra. Tetra was a high and mighty Mermaid, very mean and full of herself and to her, she was the prettiest in the whole Merworld. When she saw Geraldine she said, "Oh will you look at that, Geraldine, you clean up real good, but you are still not as beautiful as I am. I know the king will choose me today". "Uh...Tetra, he did not choose you last year, so why would he choose you today", Leslie said.

"Oh please, my dress last year was not pretty, but this time, the king will be in awe and fall in love with my beauty and my soft hair. Then he will be my own prince charming. Oh! have you noticed how pretty my hair is....", on and on Tetra went until the others rolled their eyes and left her while she was still talking. When they got to the huge palace that held all the Merfolk, there was no sitting space left at the back. For some reason, all Merfolk preferred to sit at the back of all the festival gatherings.

The girls had no choice but to sit at the front where they would be able to see clearly all that was going on. The other girls did not mind at all, it meant that they would be closer to the king, but Geraldine was concerned, she would not be able to get her precious sleep.

The festival had not even started, yet Geraldine was fast asleep. The back of her head was resting on the arm of the chair, and she was slumped all the way down. The festival finally begun and the King arrived. All the Mermaids except Geraldine sat up immediately and put on their best smiles. Geraldine was too busy sleeping to even notice that the king had come.

The king, on the other hand, was looking at all the maidens as he sat on his throne. "They all look the same. I don't like any of them", he whispered to his attendant. He was about to return to watching the great dancers when he caught sight of a lady, at least that was what he thought she was, fast asleep and almost falling off her chair. He smiled as she watched her, "She is a pretty one", he thought.

When the event was over, the king watched as the lady's friends tried to rouse her. He could not help but laugh as she screamed and fell off the chair. She gave her friends a mean look and got up sleepily, then she yawned and stretched and said, "Can we go now?"

They all agreed to leave, and they were about to when the king's attendant approached and told Geraldine that the king would like to see her. Geraldine was shocked, "Uh..Me?...What do you mean, the king wants to see me? I did not cause any trouble; I was asleep all the way through. Is he mad that I fell asleep? Surely he can't be". The attendant calmed her down, and he held her as they swam to meet the king.

She talked with the king for some time, and when she returned, she told her friends that the king had requested to see her the next day. All her friends were happy. "Soon we could all be friends with a Merqueen!" Leslie said, and they all clapped their hands in delight. They walked home feeling glad, but Tetra was sad and was so jealous that the king had picked Geraldine and she stormed off the palace.

Geraldine was happy about this, even her mom was much more joyful. They hoped that the next day would be a good day, but they were wrong, Tetra was too angry to let all this go so well.

At night, she snuck out of her house and acted as one of the palace maids to steal the King's necklace. She smiled evilly as she swam back home. The next morning, Tetra woke up very early and went to hide at the entrance of Geraldine's house, unhappy. Immediately Geraldine came out, she swam to her and hugged her warmly. She told her that she was delighted that the king had chosen her! But when Geraldine was not looking, she hid the necklace in her blouse.

The king was angry when Geraldine arrived, and he got even more upset when the necklace fell out of Geraldine's blouse as she bowed to greet him. Geraldine was confused and tried to explain that she had not stolen it, but the king would not hear it and he asked that she be locked up! The news spread fast till all Merfolk heard of it.

Merfolk from far and wide came to the palace, they all disagreed that Geraldine could do such a thing and they asked for an investigation. One after the other, the Merfolk were questioned until one of the guards said, "Oh wait, I saw this Mermaid leave the palace last night with a necklace in her hands", one of the guards said. The king immediately ordered that Tetra be taken away to the dungeons and kept there.

Some weeks later, all the Merfolk came together again, this time to see the king get married. It was a great occasion, the king took his wife, and they lived happily ever after!

www.ingramcontent.com/pod-product-compliance
Lightning Source LLC
Chambersburg PA
CBHW081158020426
42333CB00020B/2543